E. Hanisch, M. Kitajima, T. Wehrmann, and A. Encke (Eds.)
Endoscopic Gastric Surgery

W0043207

Springer
Berlin
Heidelberg
New York
Barcelona
Hongkong
London
Mailand
Paris
Singapur
Tokio

E. Hanisch, M. Kitajima, T. Wehrmann,
and A. Encke (Eds.)

Endoscopic Gastric Surgery

With 103 Figures in 129 Parts and 16 Tables

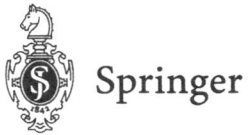 Springer

Prof. Dr. Dr. E. Hanisch, Klinik für Allgemein- und Gefäßchirurgie
Klinikum der Johann-Wolfgang-Goethe-Universität
Theodor-Stern-Kai 7, 60590 Frankfurt am Manin

Prof. Dr. M. Kitajima, F. A. C. S., Department of Surgery
Keio University School of Medicine
35 Shinanomachi, Shinjuku-k Tokyo, Japan 160

PD Dr. T. Wehrmann, Medizinische Klinik II
Zentrum für Innere Medizin, Abt. Gastroenterologie
Klinikum der Johann-Wolfgang-Goethe-Universität
Theodor-Stern-Kai 7, 60590 Frankfurt am Main

Prof. Dr. A. Encke, F. A. C. S., Klinik für Allgemein- und Gefäßchirurgie
Klinikum der Johann-Wolfgang-Goethe-Universität
Theodor-Stern-Kai 7, 60590 Frankfurt am Main

ISBN-13: 978-3-642-64045-2   e- ISBN-13: 978-3-642-59602-5
DOI: 10.1007/978-3-642-59602-5

Cataloguing-in-Publication Data applied for
Die Deutsche Bibliothek – CIP-Einheitsaufnahme
Endoscopic gastric surgery: with 16 tables / E. Hanisch ... (ed.). – Berlin ; Heidelberg ;
New York ; Barcelona ; Hongkong ; London ; Mailand ; Paris ; Singapur ; Tokyo ;
Springer 2000.
ISBN-13: 978-3-642-64045-2

© Springer-Verlag Berlin Heidelberg 2000
Softcover reprint of the hardcover 1st edition 2000

Cover Design: Frido Steinen-Broo, Barcelona
Typesetting: FotoSatz Pfeifer GmbH, D-82166 Gräfelfing
SPIN: 10673790   24/3135 – 5 4 3 2 1 0

Preface

Laparoscopy has revolutionized the world of surgery. Since the first laparoscopic cholecystectomy, minimally invasive procedures have permeated all surgical specialities.

This monograph focuses on and summarizes laparoscopic gastric operations on the basis of solid pathophysiological considerations, while carefully weighing surgical options against medical therapies. Thus, fundoplication, an almost forgotten surgical procedure, has now gained widespread acceptance, an acceptance which is ever increasing in the face of economic pressure.

The same is true of cardiomyotomy for achalasia. Surgery for morbid obesity, laparoscopically performed, has almost completely replaced the open procedure, not only because the postoperative recovery of patients is so remarkable, but also because weight loss is dramatic and sustained. Nevertheless, it should be borne in mind that this kind of operation has a steep learning curve and should only be carried out by surgeons with extensive experience of laparoscopic techniques. Assistant sessions with colleagues already familiar with the operation are to be highly recommended. Even more demanding are gastric resections and gastrectomies.

Of course, in malignant disease of the stomach, pro and contra arguments are also emerging with respect to the problem of port site metastases. Experience with laparoscopic colorectal surgery to date has provided no evidence of an increased incidence of port site metastases. Most evidently these are to be explained by technical insufficiencies i.e. tumor laceration during the procedure or extraction of the specimen.

Moreover, oncological standards can be clearly adhered to laparoscopically. Definite oncological results from clinical studies, however, have to be awaited.

Certainly, laparoscopic gastric surgery, including fundoplication, cardiomyotomy, and banding, is only in its infancy. It is our hope, therefore, that this monograph will stimulate further development, particularly in these areas.

E. Hanisch, Frankfurt, M. Kitajima, Tokyo,
T. Wehrmann, Frankfurt, A. Encke, Frankfurt

Contents

1 Gastroesophageal Reflux Disease
T. Wehrmann 1

2 Laparoscopic Antireflux Surgery in
Gastroesophageal Reflux Disease (GERD)
E. Hanisch, T.C. Schmandra, and A. Encke 23

3 Achalasia: Pathophysiology, Diagnosis, and
Nonoperative Treatment
T. Wehrmann and T. Schmitt 35

4 Laparoscopic Cardiomyotomy for Achalasia
E. Hanisch, T.C. Schmandra, and A. Encke 56

5 Pathogenetic Aspects of Obesity
T. Konrad 61

6 Adjustable Silicone Gastric Banding
E. Hanisch, T.C. Schmandra, and A. Encke 73

7 Totally Laparoscopic Distal Gastrectomy
with Extended Lymph Node Dissection
I. Uyama, A. Sugioka, J. Fujita, and A. Hasumi 87

8 Laparoscopic Surgery for Early Gastric Cancer:
Lesion-Lifting Method and Intragastric Mucosal
Resection
M. Ohgami, Y. Otani, T. Furukawa, K. Kumai,
T. Kubota, J. Tokuyama, Y.-I. Kim, and M. Kitajima . 97

9 Laparoscopic Gastric Resection and Gastrectomy
E. Bärlehner 112

Subject Index 133

Contributors

E. Bärlehner, Dr., Klinikum Berlin-Buch, Surgical Clinic,
Hobrechtsfelder Chaussee 100, D-13125 Berlin, Germany

A. Encke, Prof. Dr., F. A. C. S., Klinik für Allgemein- und
Gefäßchirurgie, Klinikum der J.W. Goethe-Universität,
Theodor-Stern-Kai 7, 60590 Frankfurt am Main, Germany

J. Fujita, Dr., Department of Surgery, Fujita Health
University, School of Medicine, 1-98 Dengakugakubo,
Kutsukake-cho, Toyoake, 470-1192, Aichi, Japan

T. Furukawa, Dr., Department of Surgery, Keio University
School of Medicine, 35 Shinanomachi, Shinjuku-K Tokyo,
Japan 160

E. Hanisch, Prof. Dr. Dr., Klinik für Allgemein- und
Gefäßchirurgie, Klinikum der J.W. Goethe-Universität,
Theodor-Stern-Kai 7, 60590 Frankfurt am Main, Germany

A. Hasumi, Dr., Department of Surgery, Fujita Health
University, School of Medicine, 1-98 Dengakugakubo,
Kutsukake-cho, Toyoake, 470-1192, Aichi, Japan

Y.-I. Kim, Dr., Department of Surgery, Keio University
School of Medicine, 35 Shinanomachi, Shinjuku-K Tokyo,
Japan 160

M. Kitajima, Dr., F.A.C.S., Department of Surgery,
Keio University School of Medicine, 35 Shinanomachi,
Shinjuku-K Tokyo, Japan 160

T. Konrad, Dr., Medizinische Klinik I, J.W.-Goethe-
Universität, Theodor-Stern-Kai 7, 60590 Frankfurt am
Main, Germany

T. Kubota, Dr., Department of Surgery, Keio University
School of Medicine, 35 Shinanomachi, Shinjuku-K Tokyo,
Japan 160

K. Kumai, Dr., Department of Surgery, Keio University
School of Medicine, 35 Shinanomachi, Shinjuku-K Tokyo,
Japan 160

M. Ohgami, Dr., Department of Surgery, Keio University
School of Medicine, 35 Shinanomachi, Shinjuku-K Tokyo,
Japan 160

Y. Otani, Dr., Department of Surgery, Keio University
School of Medicine, 35 Shinanomachi, Shinjuku-K Tokyo,
Japan 160

T. C. Schmandra, Dr., Klinik für Allgemein- und
Gefäßchirurgie, Klinikum der J.W. Goethe-Universität,
Theodor-Stern-Kai 7, 60590 Frankfurt am Main, Germany

T. Schmitt, Dr., Medizinische Klinik II,
J.W. Goethe-Universität, Theodor-Stern-Kai 7,
60590 Frankfurt am Main, Germany

A. Sugioka, Dr., Department of Surgery, Fujita Health
University, School of Medicine, 1-98 Dengakugakubo,
Kutsukake-cho, Toyoake, 470-1192, Aichi, Japan

J. Tokuyama, Dr., Department of Surgery, Keio University
School of Medicine, 35 Shinanomachi, Shinjuku-K Tokyo,
Japan 160

I. Uyama, Dr., Department of Surgery, Fujita Health
University, School of Medicine, 1–98 Dengakugakubo,
Kutsukake-cho, Toyoake, 470-1192, Aichi, Japan

T. Wehrmann, PD Dr., Medizinische Klinik II,
J.W. Goethe-Universität, Theodor-Stern-Kai 7,
60590 Frankfurt am Main, Germany

CHAPTER 1

Gastroesophageal Reflux Disease

T. Wehrmann

Introduction and Definitions

Gastroesophageal reflux is a multifactorial process and most often a normal physiological event. When acid reflux causes symptoms or physical complications, we have gastroesophageal reflux disease (GERD). Some patients, however, may experience symptoms even at physiological levels of reflux ("irritable esophagus"). GERD is the most common disease of the esophagus and one of the most prevalent conditions involving the alimentary tract.

The term "reflux esophagitis" refers to mucosal damage, such as epithelial erosions or ulcerations accompanied by inflammation. However, the majority of patients with symptomatic GERD have no endoscopic evidence of esophagitis.

A sliding hiatus hernia (cephalad displacement of the stomach wall at its junction into the thorax by a distance of > 2 cm) is often present in patients with GERD, but most subjects with hiatus hernia do not suffer from symptomatic reflux.

In some patients with chronic esophagitis, the distal esophageal mucosa will be replaced by specialized columnar epithelium resembling intestinal mucosa. This esophageal epithelial metaplasia of variable length is called Barrett's esophagus and bears a considerable risk for the development of dysplasia and carcinoma.

Epidemiology

Symptomatic reflux is a common problem. It is more common in the elderly (> 40 years) and seems to be a Western trait (Holloway and Orenstein 1991). Since heartburn is the classic symptom of GERD (see below), it often serves as a marker for GERD in epidemiological studies.

A survey carried out among 355 hospital employees revealed that up to 15% experienced heartburn at least once a month (Wienbeck and Barnet 1989). In another survey, 200 of 800 randomly questioned adults reported attacks of heartburn at least once a month. While 40% of the patients took antacids for their heartburn, however, only a quarter sought medical advice from their physicians (Locke et al. 1997; Pace et al. 1991).

Whilst excessive reflux of gastric acid causes esophagitis, only 30% – 79% of patients revealed esophagitis at endoscopy (Johnsson et al. 1987; Loof et al. 1993). It was proposed that only 10% of GERD patients will develop esophagitis, that 10% of patients with esophagitis will develop Barrett's esophagus, and that in nearly 10% of patients with Barrett's metaplasia, esophageal adenocarcinoma will occur ("Ten percent rule").

GERD affected males and females equally, but there seems to be a preponderance of males among the patients who develop esophagitis (2.5:1) and Barrett's esophagus. Although GERD does not significantly affect life expectancy, it can impair quality of life and GERD-associated complications may be responsible for considerable morbidity (Keller et al. 1995; Kuster et al. 1994; McDougall et al. 1996; Schindlbeck et al. 1992; Trimble et al. 1995).

Pathophysiology

Winkelstein (1935) first suggested that GERD and esophagitis were related to the digestive action of gastric juices on the esophageal mucosa. Since then, theories of the pathophysiologic background of reflux disease have undergone continuous evolution. Even in 1960, it was still believed that GERD was primarily the consequence of a sliding hiatus hernia. Later on, attention was focused on the lower esophageal sphincter (LES) and the belief that an abnormally low LES resting pressure was the major culprit in GERD. Nowadays, there is consensus that the excessive exposure of the esophageal mucosa to gastric acid results from several factors. These pathopysiological factors responsible for GERD include a defective reflux barrier of the LES, a weak clearance function of the tubular esophagus, a delayed gastric emptying, a decreased resistance of the esophageal mucosa, and a highly aggressive potency of the refluxate. A recent multivariate analysis of risk factors for esophagitis indicates that the impaired esophageal acid clearance and the defective LES function are the two major independent causes of GERD (Cadiot et al. 1997).

Lower Esophageal Sphincter Dysfunction

Interposed between the positive intraabdominal pressure and the negative intrathoracic pressure, the LES serves as the main reflux barrier at the gastroesophageal junction. Due to a combined tonic activity of the distal esophageal smooth muscles, the smooth muscle fibers from the gastric fundus, and the pinchcock-like activity of the crural diaphragm, the LES generates a nearly 2–5-cm long high pressure zone (normal resting pressure between 10–35 mmHg). Although this region can be easily identified by manometric studies (Fig. 1.1), it is not a distinct anatomic sphincter.

The LES resting tone varies throughout the day and night, particularly as a consequence of food ingestion. Therefore, a single LES pressure measurement did not reflect accurately the LES function (Dent et al. 1988).

Gastroesophageal reflux occurs mainly during episodes of very weak LES pressure (< 4 mmHg). This is the case during swallow-induced LES

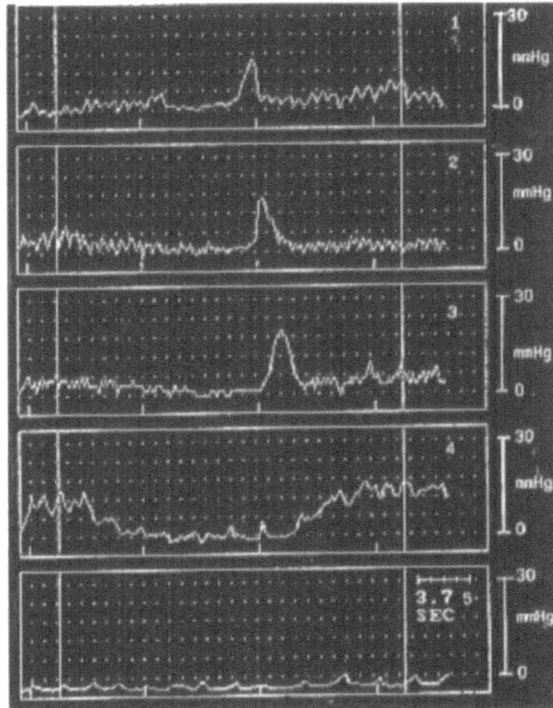

Fig. 1.1. Lower esophageal sphincter relaxation during swallowing demonstrated by esophageal manometry

relaxation (Fig. 1.1) and the so-called transient sphincter relaxations. These transient LES relaxations are usually of longer duration (5–30 s) than swallow-induced relaxations, are not accompanied by tubular esophageal peristaltic activity, are virtually absent during sleep, and were provoked by gastric fundus distention via a vago-vagally mediated reflex. Nearly all reflux episodes in healthy subjects and about two thirds of the episodes in patients with GERD were the consequence of these transient LES relaxations. Consequently, free reflux of gastric contents through a hypotonic basal LES pressure (<10 mmHg) accounts for only one third of the reflux episodes in patients with GERD. Due to the short duration (<4 s) of swallow-induced LES relaxations (and simultaneous esophageal peristaltic activity), they were not usually accompanied by significant gastroesophageal reflux (Freidin et al. 1991; Holloway and Dent 1990; Holloway et al. 1991; Mittal and McCallum 1988; Mittal et al. 1989; Sifrim et al. 1996).

However, until today, the exact reason why the number of transient sphincter relaxations is increased, and the basal LES pressure is weakened in patients with GERD, is completely unknown (Mittal and Balaban 1997).

Hiatus Hernia

The over-representation of a sliding hiatus hernia (Fig. 1.2) in patients with reflux esophagitis suggests a causal relationship, although the exact nature of the relationship is currently unclear. It has been proposed that

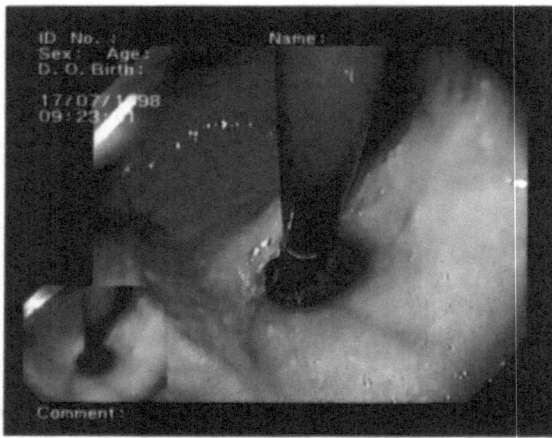

Fig. 1.2. Hiatus hernia seen on endoscopy

the hiatus hernia may act as a fluid trap permitting the re-reflux of gastric contents from the hernia sac during swallowing. This process may be repeated with subsequent swallows.

Furthermore, the displacement of the LES into the chest may alter sphincter competence. It has been shown that extrinsic compression of the gastroesophageal junction by the crural diaphragm and positive intraabdominal pressure significantly enhance the LES barrier function (Mittal and Balaban 1997; Mittal et al. 1989). Both factors will be lost in the case of a hiatus hernia.

Increased Intraabdominal Pressure

Another non-sphincteric mechanism affecting the degree of acid reflux is the pressure gradient across the gastroesophageal junction. This gradient favors reflux and is resisted by the basal LES tone. Therefore, an increase in intraabdominal pressure (for example during pregnancy or in severely obese patients) magnifies this gradient and tends to promote reflux.

Impaired Esophageal Acid Clearance

When reflux occurs, the efficiency with which the refluxate is cleared is the major determinant of the duration of esophageal acid exposure. This esophageal acid clearance is a two-step process: Firstly, the gastric volume is removed by peristaltic activity (and occasionally by gravity) and, thereafter, the residual acid is neutralized by swallowed saliva. Both factors may be impaired in reflux disease (Dodds et al. 1990; Corraziari et al. 1986).

Peristaltic dysfunction (Fig. 1.3) had been found in 25% of patients with "mild" esophagitis, but could be detected in more than half of patients with severe esophagitis (Kahrilas et al. 1986). Especially patients with scleroderma (who had markedly impaired distal esophageal peristaltic activity) tend to have severe esophagitis and are very likely to develop GERD-related complications (i.e., strictures or ulcers) (Wehrmann and Caspary 1990). It has been shown that the acid clearance time is inversely related to the rate of intact primary peristalsis, whereas secondary peristalsis seems to be of minor importance (Dodds et al. 1990).

The diminished esophageal motor function in patients with GERD could not be reverted to normal following either effective medical or

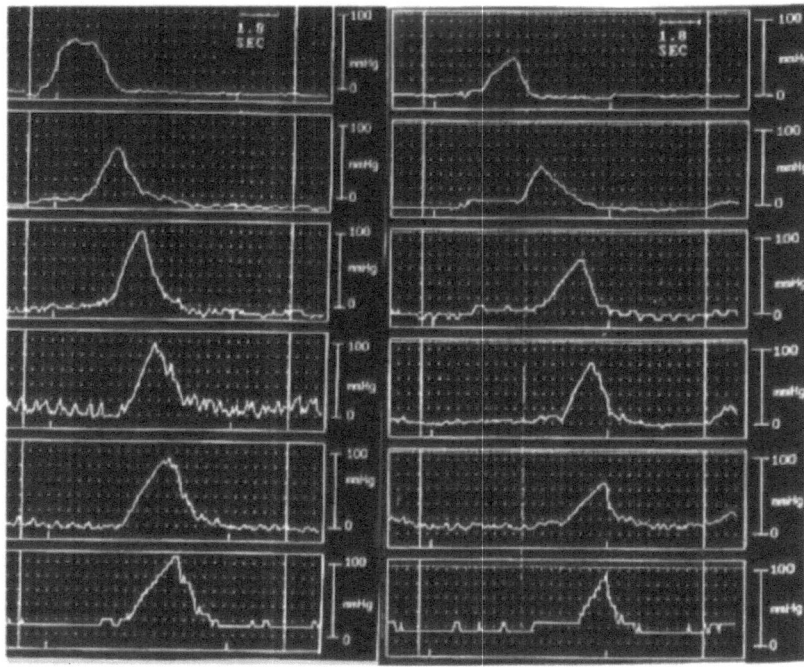

Fig. 1.3. Distal esophageal motility in health (*left*) and reflux disease (*right*; mano-metric findings)

surgical therapy. However, the question of whether impaired peristaltic function is a primary defect in GERD (and not induced by inflammatory esophageal damage), remains controversial.

Saliva is the second essential factor required for normal esophageal acid clearance. It has a pH of 6–8 and is, therefore, a relative base compared with the acid gastric juice. Spontaneous swallowing results in a saliva production of about 0.5 ml/min. The contribution of impaired salivary function to abnormal acid clearance, however, has received little attention. The rate of salivation in patients with GERD did not seem to differ from normal controls, but in patients with severe esophagitis a blunted salivary response had been proposed (Holloway and Orenstein 1991). Furthermore, diminished salivation during sleep explains why nocturnal reflux events are associated with prolonged acid clearance times. Consequently, patients with xerostomia showed dramatically delayed esophageal acid clearance and higher grades of esophagitis.

Also, cigarette smokers have hyposalivation which prolongs esophageal acid clearance; thus, cigarette smoking tends to favor gastroesophageal reflux (which was traditionally believed to be due to a lowering effect of nicotine on the LES) (Kahrilas and Gupta 1990).

Impaired Esophageal Mucosal Resistance

Because not all patients with GERD develop esophagitis, it can be speculated that the esophageal mucosa has its own resistance capacity. Mucus, bicarbonate ions, and the unstirred water layer may contribute to this mucosal resistance. The mucus has gel-like properties which serve as a barrier to large molecules such as pepsin. Although hydrogen ions can enter the mucus layer, they can be neutralized by bicarbonate ions within the unstirred water layer. Furthermore, the stratified squamous epithelial cells and their tight intercellular junctions are initially impermeable for hydrogen ions. However, to preserve this protective mechanism, optimal mucosal blood flow and regular epithelial cell replication is mandatory (Orlando 1996).

Delayed Gastric Emptying

The occurrence of reflux depends on the reservoir of gastric contents. The gastric volume is mainly determined by the amount of oral intake, the rate of gastric emptying, the volume of gastric acid secretion, and the amount of duodeno-gastric reflux (Holloway and Orenstein 1991). Moreover, excessive gastric (fundus) distention exaggerates transient LES relaxations, and therefore directly promotes gastroesophageal reflux (Holloway et al. 1991; Wyman et al. 1990).

Older scintigraphic studies had demonstrated delayed gastric emptying of solids in nearly half of all patients with reflux esophagitis. However, since these studies had several methodological drawbacks, recent investigations suggest that delayed gastric emptying promotes acid reflux only in a small subset (about 10%) of patients with GERD (McCallum et al. 1981). Nevertheless, several studies demonstrated the usefulness of gastroprokinetics (which mainly stimulate gastric emptying) in the medical therapy of GERD (see below).

Gastric Acid Hypersecretion and Duodeno-gastric Reflux

The majority of patients with GERD have normal levels of gastric acid output, and thus it is generally believed that this factor is not important in determing the severity of acid reflux. However, recent studies suggest the possibility that GERD patients not responding to conventional antisecretory drug therapy may have higher rates of gastric acid secretion than normal controls (Collen et al. 1990). Especially in patients with Barrett's esophagus, two studies demonstrated higher rates of gastric basal acid output than in healthy subjects. Another series, however, did not support these findings of abnormal acid secretion in patients with Barrett's mucosa (Hirschowitz 1991). A recent multivariate analysis detected that the peak acid output may be an independent risk factor in patients with GERD to develop reflux esophagitis (Cadiot et al. 1997).

Reflux of duodenal contents (especially bile salts) into the stomach and esophagus has long been suspected to be of etiological relevance for esophagitis. This hypothesis is supported by the fact that bile salts act synergistically with acids in causing esophageal mucosal damage. However, the precise role of duodeno-gastroesophageal reflux in GERD remains controversial. Whereas some studies demonstrated higher amounts of bile salts in the refluxate of patients with esophagitis or Barrett's mucosa, others did not. Techniques for accurate prolonged monitoring of duodenogastric reflux (spectrophotometric bilirubin measurement, sodium ion electrode measurement) have been developed only just recently, and the results from ongoing trials (using these new technologies) have to be awaited (DeCaestacker 1997).

Diagnosis

Clinical Presentation

Heartburn is the classic symptom of GERD. The retrosternal burning may radiate into the epigastrium, the neck, the throat, and occasionally the back. Frequently, it occurs postprandially, particularly after consumption of fatty meals, spicy food, citrus fruits, chocolate, or alcohol. Heartburn may be also aggravated in recumbence or by bending over. The daily presence of heartburn and acid regurgitation have a positive predictive value for reflux esophagitis of nearly 60%.

Other GERD-associated symptoms are listed in Table 1.1. The presence of dysphagia can indicate the development of a peptic stricture.

Table 1.1. Symptomatic presentation of gastro-esophageal reflux disease

Esophageal	Pharyngeal	Pulmonary
Heartburn	Chronic cough	Asthma
Epigastric pain	Hoarseness	Chronic cough
Acid regurgitation	Globus sensation	
Dysphagia	Throat pain	
Odynophagia		

This usually occurs in the setting of long-standing heartburn with slowly progressive dysphagia for solids, followed by liquids, and a moderate loss of weight. Otherwise, an adenocarcinoma in a patient with Barrett's esophagus may cause (more rapidly developing) dysphagia. However, some patients with GERD lack specific symptoms and their disease is discovered incidentally, e.g., erosive esophagitis or Barrett's metaplasia during endoscopy for malabsorption problems. In particular, patients with Barrett's esophagus may present with adenocarcinoma as their first and only manifestation of GERD. The exact reason why GERD can be present with or without symptoms is not fully understood.

Gastroesophageal reflux may also present with complaints not immediately referable to the gastrointestinal tract, featuring chest pain, respiratory symptoms, or ear, nose, and throat (ENT) problems (Table 1.1). Asthma may be triggered by direct microaspiration of gastric acid or via a vagally mediated bronchospasm triggered by intraesophageal acid exposure (Simpson 1995).

Endoscopy

Esophagoscopy is the first-line procedure for evaluating patients with suspected GERD. It permits a verification of reflux esophagitis and detection of GERD-associated conditions (like hiatus hernia) or complications (Barrett's mucosa, esophageal ulcer, peptic stricture, carcinoma). Erosive esophagitis is the hallmark finding in GERD and it enables an assessment of the severity of reflux disease (Figs. 1.4 and 1.5). The endoscopic findings can be graded according to the Savary–Miller (Savary and Miller 1978) (Table 1.2) or the MUSE classification (Table 1.3). Up to now, the Savary–Miller classification is in more widespread use, but this grading system has the disadvantage of (falsely) suggesting Barrett's esophagus and peptic strictures as more advanced grades of esophagitis.

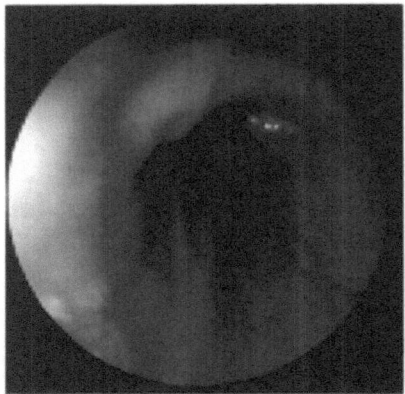

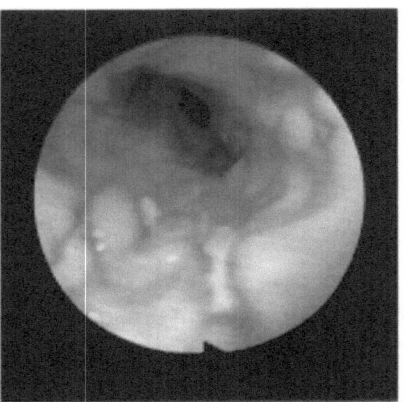

Fig. 1.4. Reflux esophagitis grade I (endoscopic presentation)

Fig. 1.5. Reflux esophagitis grade III (endoscopic presentation)

Degree	Endoscopic findings
I.	Singular erosions
II.	Semi-circumferential erosions
III.	Circumferential erosions
IV.	Peptic esophageal stricture
	Peptic esophageal ulcer
	Barrett's metaplasia

Table 1.2. Classification of reflux esophagitis according to Savary and Miller (1978)

Table 1.3. Classification of reflux disease according to the MUSE-system

Degree	Metaplasia	Ulcer	Stricture	Erosion
0	None	None	None	None
1	1 Tongue	Savary ulcer	>9 mm	Singular
2	≥2 Tongues	Barrett ulcer	≥9 mm	Semi-circumferential
3	Circumferential	Combined ulcer	Stricture + brachyesophagus	Circumferential

The precise role of histology in the diagnosis of GERD is not completely clear. The presence of a neutrophil infiltrate in the lamina propria is generally believed to be a specific marker for esophagitis, but it is very insensitive and, therefore, can also be found in at least 20% of normal

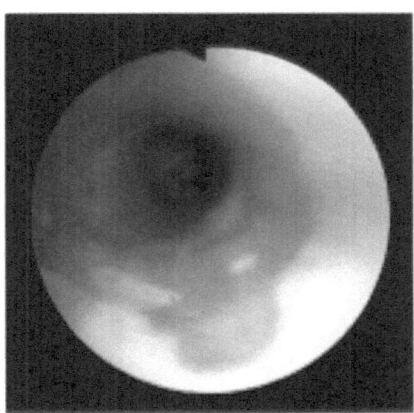

Fig. 1.6. Barrett's esophagus (endoscopic appearance)

subjects. It had been demonstrated that histologic findings did not accurately enable the detection of patients with pathological reflux (on 24-h
pH-metry) when esophagitis is not present at endoscopy. However,
biopsy is the major clue to diagnosing Barrett's esophagus and associated dysplasia. If Barrett's esophagus is suspected endoscopically
(Fig. 1.6), multiple four-quadrant biopsies have to be obtained. Patients
with histologically proven Barrett's segment (of any length) should
undergo endoscopic follow-up (Provenzale et al. 1994). The diagnosis of
Barrett's segment with dysplasia should not be made if active esophagitis is simultaneously present. These patients must undergo intensive
medical treatment with endoscopic reexamination before entertaining a
definite diagnosis of dysplasia. In the case of low-grade dysplasia, endoscopic surveillance with repeated examinations every 3–6 months is
mandatory. If high-grade dysplasia has been confirmed by two independent experienced pathologists, the patient should be treated either surgically (esophagectomy) or endoscopically (mucosectomy, photody-
namic laser ablation).

Radiology

In general, radiology plays no significant role in the managment of
reflux disease. Many patients do not have esophagitis and will be
expected to have a normal barium esophagogram. When compared with
endoscopy, the radiographic sensitivity to detect moderate or severe
esophagitis has been reported to be as high as 90% (Ott et al. 1986).

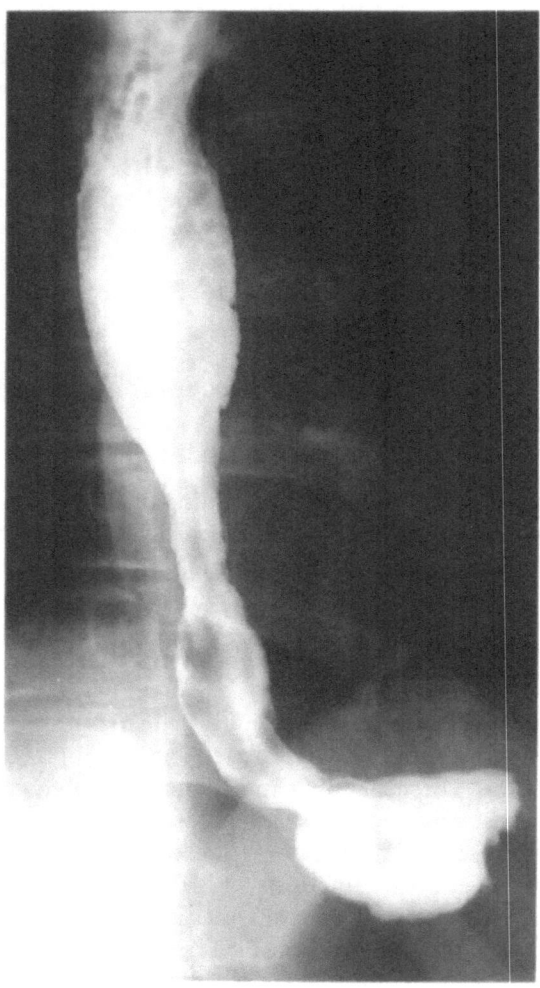

Fig. 1.7. Peptic esophageal stricture (radio-
graphic presentation)

Using double-contrast techniques, thickened longitudinal walls, thickening of the esophageal wall, and mucosal irregularities indicated esophagitis. Peptic strictures can also be clearly depicted (Fig. 1.7). However, the sensitivity to detect Barrett's mucosa is very low. The presence
of a sliding hiatus hernia, which could be accurately diagnosed by radi-
ography, did not indicate GERD, since it may be present in up to 40% of
normal subjects. Modern radiographic techniques, such as spiral computed tomography (CT), have until yet no special role in the manage-

ment of GERD. Future developments in the field of virtual endoscopy (based on spiral CT) may change this situation.

Esophageal pH-Metry

Ambulatory 24-h intraesophageal pH-monitoring has now become the technique of choice and the diagnostic "gold standard" for the detection of reflux disease. Nevertheless, it should not be considered as a perfect "gold standard" for diagnosing GERD (since up to 20% of patients with erosive esophagitis may have normal findings at pH-monitoring), it is the only means to identify the large number of reflux patients without esophagitis (Tytgat et al. 1989).

For intraesophageal pH-metry, a 1.8-mm thin probe has to be inserted transnasally and placed 5 cm above the (manometrically identified) LES (Fig. 1.8). The pH data were collected in a small, lightweight box worn on

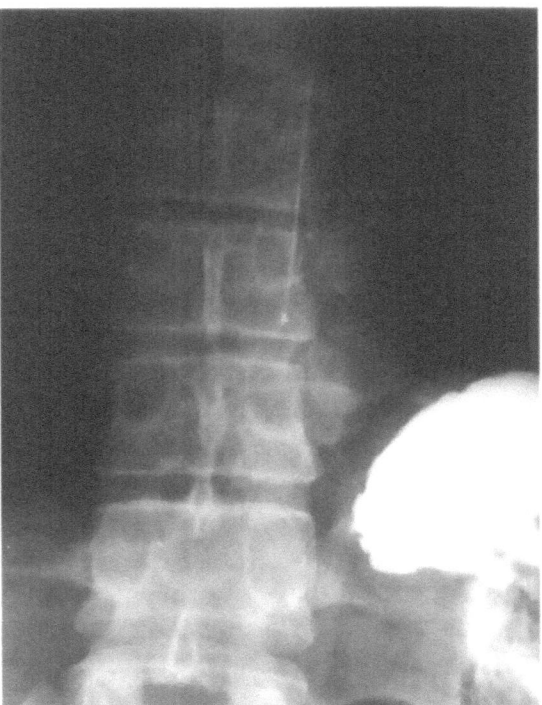

Fig. 1.8. Placement of intraesophageal pH-metry probe (radiographic presentation)

a waist belt. Routinely, pH-recording was prolonged over 24 h and the stored data were analyzed by personal computer. The examinations were performed on an outpatient basis without any dietary restrictions.

Multiple parameters can be obtained from the 24-h pH-recordings (Table 1.4). Those used more often are the percentage of time with a pH < 4, the number of all reflux episodes (with pH < 4), the number of long lasting (> 5 min) reflux episodes, and the duration of the longest reflux episode, respectively. In general, patients with GERD exhibit a higher number of acid reflux episodes and a prolonged acid exposure than

Table 1.4. Intraesophageal pH-monitoring (24-h). Parameters and normal values (data from literature)

Parameter	Cheadle (Dundee)	DeMeester (Omaha)	Masclee (Leiden)	Mattioli (Bologna)	Wehrmann (Frankfurt)	Weiser (Munich)
Subjects (n)	50	50	27	20	30	31
pH <4% of total time	2.1	1.5	1.7	1.9	1.8	2.0
pH <4% upright time	3.0	2.3	2.6	2.8	2.7	2.8
pH <4% supine time	1.0	0.6	0.0	0.7	1.0	0.7
RE per 24 h (n)	11	19	18	25	50	23
Longest RE (min)	6.4	6.7	6.3	5.2	6.0	–
RE >5 min/h (n)	0.72	0.84	–	0.03	<1	1

RE, reflux episodes; –, not reported.

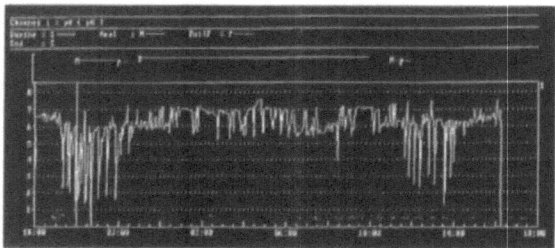

Fig. 1.9. Long-term intraesophageal pH-metry in a healthy volunteer

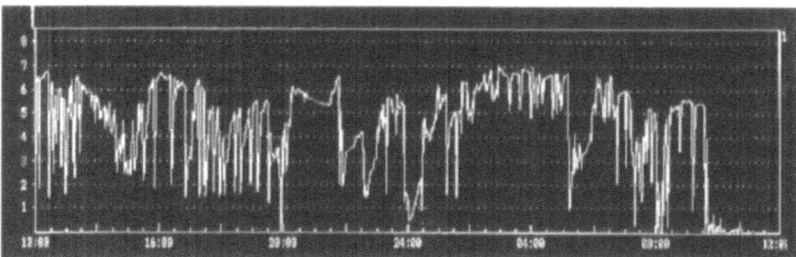

Fig. 1.10. Long-term intraesophageal pH-metry in a patient with reflux disease

healthy controls (Figs. 1.9, 1.10). In more severe cases, acid reflux may occur during the day and at night. Furthermore, ambulatory pH-monitoring allows a temporal correlation of acid reflux events with patients' complaints. Therefore, it has an important role in the assessment of atypical symptoms (chest pain, nocturnal wheezing, hoarseness, etc.) where reflux is suspected to be the cause of these symptoms.

Intraesophageal pH-metry is generally indicated in patients with typical reflux symptoms but without esophagitis, patients with atypical complaints (such as ENT problems or asthma), and patients with reflux not responding to conventional treatment (i.e., standard doses of proton-pump inhibitors). It has been shown by pH-monitoring that some patients (about 5% of reflux patients) need even higher doses of antisecretory drugs to control their excessive acid reflux (up to 120 mg of omeprazole daily).

Patients in whom antireflux surgery is intended should also undergo intraesophageal pH-metry, especially if any doubt about the diagnosis exists.

Esophageal Manometry

Esophageal manometry is of little value in the diagnosis of GERD. In the past, a lowered LES pressure (<15 mmHg) was held to be the most important pathophysiological factor in reflux disease. Nowadays, it is well known that the majority of patients with GERD will have normal LES pressures and also regular esophageal body motor function. The main indication (in the field of GERD) for esophageal manometry today is for patients in whom another diagnosis is suspected (e.g., achalasia, diffuse esophageal spasm, scleroderma), as well as for patients being considered for antireflux surgery. In patients with specific esophageal motor disorders, manometry enables a definite diagnosis to be established, and preoperative manometry is worthwhile to identify major peristaltic abnormalities which might increase the risk of postoperative dysphagia (see Fig. 1.3). With such information, the surgeon may wish to perform a "floppy" fundoplication or an incomplete wrap. In addition, manometry is used for localization of the LES prior to pH-monitoring.

Non-operative Treatment

The rationale for GERD therapy depends on a careful definition of specific goals. In patients without esophagitis, the therapeutic aim is simply to relieve acid-related symptoms. In patients with esophagitis, the ultimate goal is to heal the inflammation while attempting to prevent the development of GERD-related complications, namely strictures and Barrett's metaplasia.

These goals are set against a complex background: Reflux is a chronic disease that may wax and wane in symptom intensity, and a clear relationship between symptoms and either the amount of acid exposure or the presence of esophagitis did not exist.

Natural History

Only sparse data on the natural history of GERD exists (Locke et al. 1997; McDougall et al. 1996; Pace et al. 1991; Trimble et al. 1995; Schindlbeck et al. 1992). In general, reflux symptoms and esophagitis may wax and wane in individual patients and, therefore, GERD commonly seems not to be a chronic progressive disease. However, a recent investigation showed that nearly three quarters of patients previously diagnosed as having esophagitis still had significant morbidity related to GERD more than 10 years following diagnosis. Therefore, in those patients presenting with GERD (but without esophagitis) for the first time, medical therapy should be initiated for a limited time span. Thereafter, an on-demand medication seems to be reasonable. Continuous medical treatment (or operative treatment) may be necessary only for a very small subgroup of patients without esophagitis. In patients with esophagitis, the inflammation should first be remedied by medical treatment, but if a relapse occurs either long-term medication or surgery should be intended.

Physical Measures and Nutrition

Effective therapy for patients with only infrequent and mild heartburn is possible by lifestyle and dietary modifications. It has been shown that nocturnal reflux could be reduced by elevation of the head of the bed (Harvey et al. 1987).

Cigarette smoking can reduce LES pressure and delay esophageal acid clearance (Kahrilas and Gupta 1990). Hence, patients with GERD should stop smoking. Also, alcohol may provoke acid reflux. Many patients reported intolerance to various foods. Avoidance of these is recommended whenever possible. Meals of large volume or with high fat content may also provoke strong postprandial reflux (by gastric distention and reflectory transient LES relaxation, or by retarding gastric emptying) and, therefore, should be avoided.

Furthermore, the patient's history should be carefully evaluated for drugs that may facilitate reflux (e.g., theophylline, α-adrenergic agonists, antidepressants, nitrates, calcium channel blocking agents). However, besides the known deleterious effects of theophylline on reflux, convincing evidence that the other drugs may significantly affect esophageal acid exposure is lacking.

Medical Treatment

Because of their superior efficacy in acute and long-term treatment, proton-pump inhibitors (PPI) have become the mainstay of medical therapy for reflux esophagitis. Motility-stimulating drugs or mucosal protective agents are of importance for patients with GERD, but without esophagitis or after esophagitis has been successfully treated, for long-term maintenance therapy.

Proton-Pump Inhibitors

Substituted benzimidazoles (omeprazole, lansoprazole, pantoprazole) are potent and long-acting inhibitors of both basal and stimulated gastric acid secretion. They all act by selective, non-competitive inhibition of the $H+/K+$ adenosine triphosphatase (ATPase) enzyme located in the secretory membrane of the parietal cell. Given in standard doses (e.g., omeprazole 20 mg, lansoprazole 30 mg, pantoprazole 40 mg, all b.i.d.), they virtually ablate gastric acid secretion (> 90%) when compared with the acid reducing effect (»70%) of $H2$-antagonists (e.g., ranitidine

150 mg, b.i.d.) (Maton 1991). Controlled studies demonstrated that PPI completely abolishes reflux symptoms in the vast majority of patients with GERD during 1–2 weeks of therapy. Healing from esophagitis could be demonstrated in nearly 90% of patients after 8–12 weeks of PPI treatment. In those cases resistant to standard doses of PPI, higher doses of PPI (e.g., omeprazole 80–160 mg per day) are effective (Castell et al. 1996; Corinaldesi et al. 1995; Hetzel et al. 1988; Mössner 1995).

Several studies proved the superiority of PPI agents vs. H2-antagonists in controlling reflux symptoms and esophagitis, as well as for longterm maintenance treatment (Dehn et al. 1990; Feldman et al. 1993; Klinkenberg-Knol et al. 1987; Richter et al. 1996; Vigneri et al. 1995). Regarding efficacy and side-effects profile, the three available PPI differ very little. Since long-term treatment (1–5 years) with PPI showned a remarkably low rate of side effects, they are now permitted for maintenance treatment of reflux esophagitis in most western countries.

Prokinetic Agents

This group includes betanechol, metoclopramide, domperidone, and cisapride. However, in routine clinical practice, only cisapride has assumed a significant role in the management of GERD. The substance increases the postganglionic release of acetylcholine without any antidopaminergic effects. It has only minor side effects (headache, borborygmi, abdominal cramps, diarrhea) and is permitted for long-term use even in children. Physiological studies demonstrated that cisapride enhances the esophageal body motility, the LES resting pressure, and the rate of gastric emptying. In patients with GERD, the total number of reflux episodes and the percentage of esophageal acid exposure were significantly decreased by cisapride.

Cisapride is superior to placebo in relieving heartburn and improving esophagitis in GERD patients (Baldi et al. 1988; Richter 1993). Its efficacy is comparable to that of H2-antagonists, but cisapride revealed no such profound effects on acid reflux like proton-pump inhibitors. Therefore, in view of its good tolerability, cisapride (20 mg per day) is especially indicated for maintenance therapy of GERD (Blum et al. 1993; Tytgat et al. 1992). In higher doses (10 mg t.id. or q.i.d.), it may also be used for relieving symptoms in patients without esophagitis.

Antacids and Mucosal Protective Agents

These substances are useful for on-demand treatment of GERD patients with only mild and infrequent symptoms. Antacids work primarily by neutralizing acid for brief periods, but it has been hypothesized that they additionally have mucosal protective properties. In particular, the combination of an antacid with alginic acid was believed to form a protective coating onto the esophageal mucosal surface. However, antacids, as well as the alginate/antacid combination, are clinically significantly less effective than PPI. For treatment of reflux esophagitis, high-dose regimens of antacids (between six and eight standard doses per day) are necessary, and this dosing is not only inconvenient but also associated with significant side effects (electrolyte imbalance, obstipation or diarrhea) (Graham et al. 1987; Stanciu and Bennet 1974).

References

Baldi F, Bianci-Porro G, Dobrilla G, et al. (1988) Cisapride versus placebo in the treatment of reflux esophagitis. J Clin Gastroenterol 10:614 – 18

Blum AL, Adami B, Bouzo MH, et al. (1993) Effect of cisapride on relapse of esophagitis. A multinational, placebo-controlled trial in patients healed with an antisecretory drug. Dig Dis Sci 38:551 – 60

Cadiot G, Bruhat A, Rigaud D, et al. (1997) Multivariate analysis of pathophysiological factors in reflux oesophagitis. Gut 40:167 – 74

Castell DO, Richter JE, Robinson M, et al. (1996) Efficacy and safety of lansoprazole in the treatment of erosive reflux esophagitis. Am J Gastroenterol 91:1749 – 57

Colin-Jones DG (1989) Histamine-2-receptor antagonists in gastro-oesophageal reflux. Gut 30:1305 – 8

Collen MJ, Lewis JH, Benjamin SB (1990) Gastric acid hypersecretion in refractory gastro-esophageal reflux disease. Gastroenterology 98:654 – 61

Corinaldesi R, Valentini M, Belaiche J, et al. (1995) Pantoprazole and omeprazole in the treatment of reflux oesophagitis: a european multicentre study. Aliment Pharmacol Therap 9:667 – 71

Corraziari E, Materia E, Pozzessere C, Anzini F, Torsoli A (1986) Intraluminal pH and oesophageal motility in patients with gastro-oesophageal reflux. Digestion 35:151 – 7

DeCaestacker JS (1997) Measuring duodenogastro-oesophageal reflux (DGOR). Europ J Gastroenterol Hepatol 9:1141 – 3

Dehn TCB, Shepberd HA, Colin Jones D, Kettlewell MGW, Carroll NJH (1990) Double blind comparison of omeprazole versus cimetidine in the treatment of symptomatic erosive reflux oesophahitis assessed endoscopically, histologically, and by 24 h pH monitoring. Gut 31:509 – 13

Dent J, Holloway RH, Toouli J, Dodds WJ (1988) Mechanisms of lower oesophageal sphincter incompetence in patients with symptomatic gastro-oesophageal reflux. Gut 29:1020 – 8

Dodds WJ, Kahrilas J, Dent J, Hogan WJ, Kern MK, Arndorfer RC (1990) Analysis of spontaneous gastroesophageal reflux and esophageal acid clearance in patients with reflux esophagitis. J Gastrointest Motil 2:79–89

Feldman M, Harford WV, Fisher RS, et al. (1993) Treatment of reflux esophagitis resistant to H2-receptor antagonists with lansoprazole, a new H+/K+-Atpase inhibitor: a controlled, double-blind study. Am J Gastroenterol 88:1212–7

Fennerty MB (1996) How do you spell relief in reflux esophagitis? PPI! Gastroenterology 111:826–7

Freidin N, Fisher M, Taylor W, et al. (1991) Sleep and nocturnal acid reflux in normal subjects and patients with reflux oesophagitis. Gut 32:1275–9

Graham DY, Lanza F, Dorsch ER (1987) Symptomatic reflux esophagitis: a double blind controlled comparison of antacids and alginate. Curr Therap Res 22:652–8

Harvey RF, Hadley G, Gill TR et al. (1987) Effects of sleeping with bed-head raised and of ranitidine in patients with severe peptic esophagitis. Lancet ii:1200–3

Hetzel DJ, Dent J, Reed WD, et al. (1988) Healing and relapse of severe peptic esophagitis after treatment with omeprazole. Gastroenterology 95:903–12

Hirschowitz BI (1991) A critical analysis, with appropriate controls, of gastric acid and pepsin secretion in clinical esophagitis. Gastroenterology 101:1149–58

Holloway RD, Dent J (1990) Lower esophageal sphincter dysfunction in gastroesophageal reflux disease. Gastroenterol Clin North Am 19:1–19

Holloway RD, Orenstein SR (1991) Gastro-oesophageal reflux disease. Ball Clin Gastroenterol 5:337–70

Holloway RD, Koycan P, Dent J (1991) Provocation of transient lower esophageal sphincter relaxations by meals in patients with reflux esophagitis. Dig Dis Sci 36:1034–9

Holloway RD, Dent J, Narievala F, MacKinnon AM (1996) Relation between oesophageal acid exposure and healing of oesophagitis with omeprazole in patients with severe reflux oesophagitis. Gut 38:649–54

Johnsson F, Joelsson, Gudmundsson K, Greiff L (1987) Symptoms and endoscopic findings in the diagnosis of gastrooesophageal reflux disease. Scand J Gastroenterol 22:714–8

Kahrilas P, Gupta RR (1990) Mechanisms of acid reflux associated with cigarette smoking. Gut 31:4–10

Kahrilas PJ, Dodds WJ, Hogan WJ, Kern M, Arndorfer RC, Reece A (1986) Esophageal peristaltic dysfunction in peptic esophagitis. Gastroenterology 91:897–904

Keller M, Holtmann G, Hübner J, Gschossmann J, Guerra G, Layer P (1995) Predictors of the course of symptoms in patients with gastrooesophageal reflux. Gut 37:102 (abstract)

Klinkenberg-Knol EC, Jansen JMBJ, Festen HPM, Meuwissen SGM, Lamers CHBW (1987) Double-blind multicentre comparison of omeprazole and ranitidine in the treatment of reflux oesophagitis. Lancet i:349–51

Kuster E, Ros E, Toledo-Pimentel V, Pujol A, Bordas JM, Gande L, Pera C (1994) Predictive factors of the long term outcome in gastro-oesophageal reflux-disease: six year follow-up of 107 patients. Gut 35:8–14

Locke GR, Talley NJ, Fett SL, Zinsmeister AR, Melton LJ (1997) Prevalence and clinical spectrum of gastroesophageal reflux: a population based study in Olmsted County, Minnesota. Gastroenterology 112:1448–56

Loof L, Gutell P, Eltberg B (1993) The incidence of reflux oesophagitis. A study of the endoscopy reports from a defined catchment area in Sweden. Scand J Gastroenterol 28:113–8

Maton DJ (1991) Omeprazole. N Engl J Med 324:965–75

McCallum RW, Berkowitz DM, Lerner E (1981) Gastric emptying in patients with gastroesophageal reflux. Gastroenterology 80:285–91

McDougall NI, Johnston BT, Kee F, Collins SJA, McFarland RJ, Love AHG (1996) Natural history of reflux oesophagitis: a 10 year follow up of its effect on patient symptomatology and quality of life. Gut 38:481–6

Mittal RK, McCallum RW (1988) Characteristics and frequency of transient relaxations of the lower esophageal sphincter in patients with reflux esophagitis. Gastroenterology 95:593–9

Mittal RK, Balaban GH (1997) The esophago-gastric junction. N Engl J Med 336:924–32

Mittal RK, Rochester DF, McCallum RW (1989) Sphincteric action of the diaphragm during a relaxed LES in humans. Am J Physiol 256:6139–44

Mössner J, Hölscher AH, Herz R, Schneiders A (1995) A double-blind study of pantoprazole and omeprazole in the treatment of reflux oesophagitis: a multicentre trial. Aliment Pharmacol Therap 9:321–6

Orlando RC (1996) Why is the high-grade inhibition of gastric acid secretion afforded by proton pump inhibitors often required for healing of reflux esophagitis? An epithelial perspective. Am J Gastroenterol 91:1692–6

Ott DJ, Chen YM, Gelfand DW, Munitz HA, Wu WC (1986) Analysis of multiphasic radiological investigation for detecting reflux esophagitis. Gastrointest Radiol 11:1–6

Pace F, Santalucia F, Bianci-Porro G (1991) Natural history of gastro-oesophageal reflux disease without oesophagitis. Gut 32:845–8

Provenzale D, Kemp JA, Arroa S, Wong JB (1994) A guide for surveillance in patients with Barrett's oesophagus. Am J Gastroenterol 89:670–80

Ramirez B, Richter JE (1993) Promotility drugs in the treatment of gastro-oesophageal reflux disease. Aliment Pharmacol Therap 2:5–20

Richter JE (1993) Gastro-oesophageal reflux disease. In: Kumar D, Wingate D (eds.) An illustrated guide to gastrointestinal motility. 2nd ed. Churchill, London, pp. 496–521

Richter JE, Bradley LA, DeMeester TR (1992) Normal 24-hr ambulatory pH-values. Dig Dis Sci 37:849–56

Richter JE, Sabesin SM, Kogut DG, Kerr RM, Wruble LD, Collen MJ (1996) Omeprazole vs ranitidine or ranitidine/metoclopramide in poorly responsive symptomatic gastroesophageal reflux disease. Am J Gastroenterol 91:1766–72

Robinson M, Lanza F, Avner D, Haber M (1996) Effective maintenance treatment of reflux esophagitis with low-dose lansoprazole. Ann Intern Med 124:859–67

Savary M, Miller G (1978) The esophagus. In: Grossman AG (ed) Handbook and atlas of endoscopy. Solothurn, Switzerland, pp. 135–9

Schindlbeck NE, Klauser AG, Berghammer G, Londong W, Müller-Lissner SA (1992) Three-year follow-up of patients with gastro-oesophageal reflux disease. Gut 33:1016–9

Schnatz PF, Castell JA, Castell DO (1996) Pulmonary symptoms associated with gastroesophageal reflux: Use of ambulatory pH monitoring to diagnose and to direct therapy. Am J Gastroenterol 91:1715–19

Sifrim D, Jannssens J, Vantrappen G (1996) Transient lower esophageal sphincter relaxations and esophageal body muscular contractile response in normal humans. Gastroenterology 110:659 – 68

Simpson WG (1995) Gastroesophageal reflux and asthma. Diagnosis and management. Arch Int Med 155:798 – 803

Stanciu C, Bennet JR (1974) Alginate/antacid in the reduction of gastro-oesophageal reflux. Lancet I:109 – 10

Trimble KC, Douglas S, Pryde A, Heading RC (1995) Clinical characteristics and natural history of symptomatic but not excess gastrooesophageal reflux. Dig Dis Sci 40:1098 – 1104

Tytgat GN, Bennett JR, Dent J, Joelsson B (1989) Oesophageal pH – monitoring – normal and abnormal. Gastroenterol Int 2:141 – 9

Tytgat GN, Anker-Hansen OJ, Carling L, et al. (1992) Effect of cisapride on relapse of reflux oesophagitis, healed with an antisecretory drug. Scand J Gastroenterol 27:175 – 83

Vigneri S, Termini R, Landro G, et al. (1995) A comparison of five maintenance therapies for reflux esophagitis. N Engl J Med 333:1106 – 10

Wehrmann T, Caspary WF (1990) Influence of cisapride on esophageal motility in healthy volunteers and patients with progressive systemic sclerosis. Klin Wochenschr 68:602 – 7

Wienbeck M, Barnert J (1989) Epidemiology of reflux disease and reflux oesophagitis. Scand J Gastroenterol 24 (suppl. 156):7 – 13

Wyman JB, Dent J, Heddle R, Dodds WJ, Toouli J, Downtown J (1990) Control of belching by the lower oesophageal sphincter. Gut 31:639 – 46

Laparoscopic Antireflux Surgery in Gastroesophageal Reflux Disease (GERD)

E. Hanisch, T.C. Schmandra, and A. Encke

Indications

Current indications for surgery include:
1. Persistent gastroesophageal reflux symptoms (GER) or development of complications (stricture, ulcer, hemorrhage) under medical therapy.
2. Patient noncompliance with medical therapy.
3. Young patients who would rather have surgery than adapt their lifestyle in the manner necessary to control GER symptoms.
4. Young patients who have pulmonary disease complicated by GERD.
5. Benign Barrett's esophagus may be treated by antireflux surgery. In particular, a subgroup of patients with persistent regurgitation in spite of medical control of esophageal acid exposure could benefit from this strategy.

Contraindications

Contraindications for laparoscopic antireflux surgery include:
1. Severe chronic obstructive pulmonary disease.
2. Secondary reflux (e.g., in pregnancy, gastric motility disorders).
3. Previous upper abdominal surgery (relative).
4. Coagulopathy (e.g., in liver cirrhosis).

Techniques of Antireflux Surgery: 360° Fundoplication

The surgeon stands between the legs of the patient with two assistants on the right and left side of the patient (Fig. 2.1). An anti-Trendelenburg position is used (Fig. 2.2).

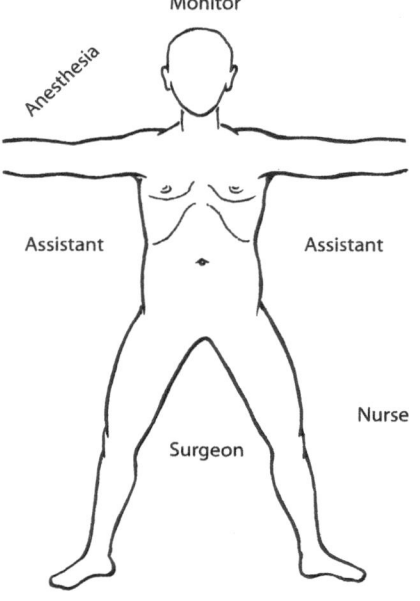

Fig. 2.1. Surgeon stands between the legs of the patient with two assistants on the right and left side

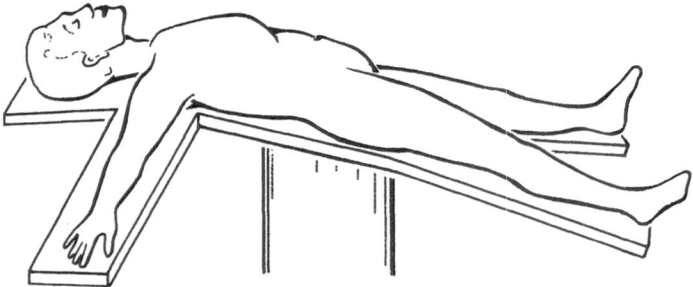

Fig. 2.2. An anti-Trendelenburg position is used

The Veress needle is introduced at the umbilicus. The pneumoperitoneum is maintained at a maximal pressure of 12 mmHg.

The camera trocar is inserted half way between the xiphoid process and the umbilicus. Three additional 12-mm trocars are placed: one

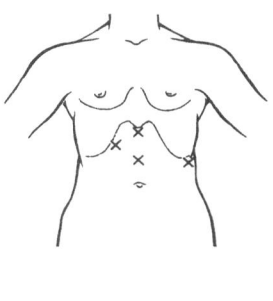

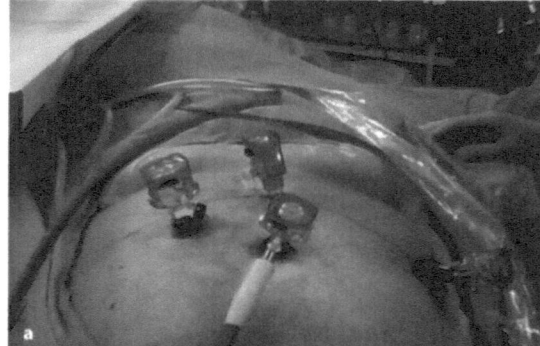

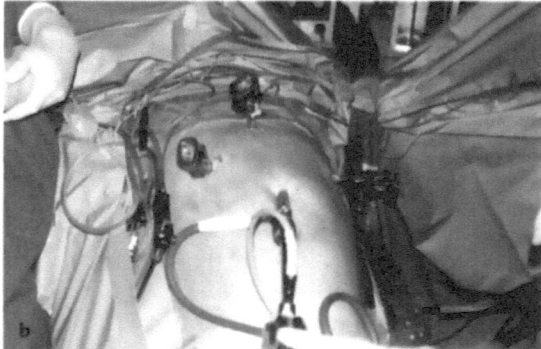

Fig. 2.3a – c. A camera trocar is inserted half way between the xiphoid process and the umbilicus. Three additional 12-mm trocars are placed: one in the midline, just below the xiphoid process, one in the right hypochondrium below the costal margin, and one in the left lateral subcostal hypochondrium

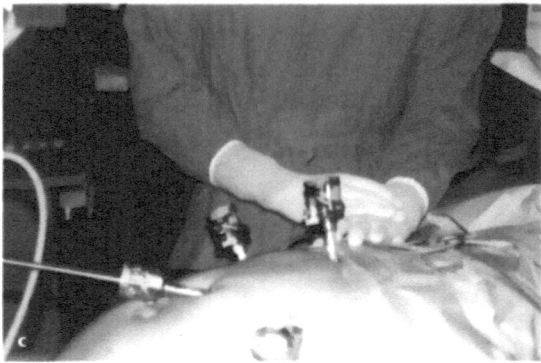

located in the midline, just below the xiphoid process, one in the right hypochondrium below the costal margin, and one in the left lateral subcostal hypochondrium (Fig. 2.3).

The left liver lobe is first lifted by a fan retractor (Auto Suture, Norwalk, Conn. USA) introduced via the subxiphoidal trocar (Fig. 2.4).

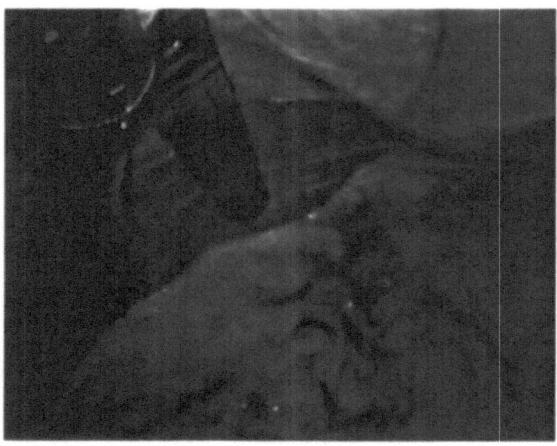

Fig. 2.4. The left liver
lobe is first lifted by a fan
retractor introduced via
the subxiphoidal trocar

The dissection starts with dividing short gastric vessels by an ultrasonic scalpel (Ultracision – Ethicon Endo-Surgery, Cincinatti, Ohio, USA) (Fig. 2.5a,b).

The fundic portion of the stomach is mobilized by this procedure, allowing it to create a loose, floppy wrap around the distal portion of the esophagus.

For a loose wrap it is also necessary to dissect the dorsal portion of the fundus (Fig. 2.6)

Next, the left and right crus are identified and a window behind the esophagus is opened by blunt dissection (Fig. 2.7a–d) (using a Hourlay Autostatic Retractor, Duchateau/Rouvreux, Belgium).

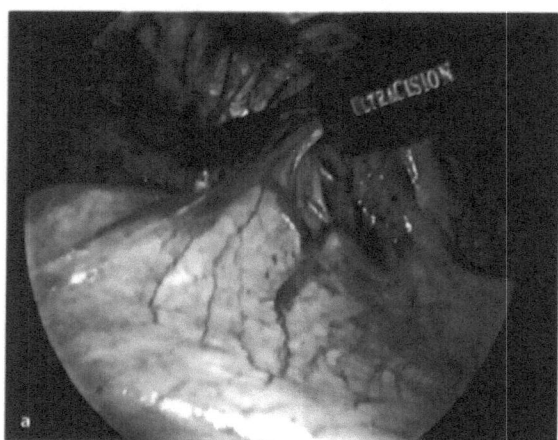

Fig. 2.5a,b. The dissection starts with dividing
short gastric vessels by
the Ultracision (Ethicon)

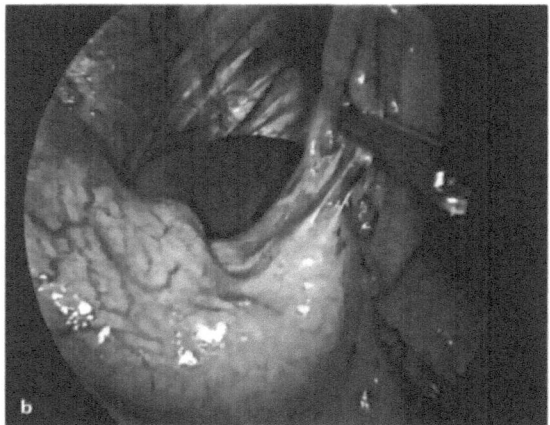

Fig. 2.5b

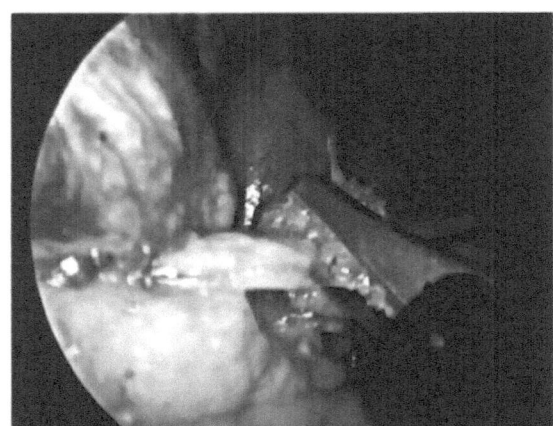

Fig. 2.6. For a loose wrap, it is also necessary to dissect the dorsal portion of the fundus

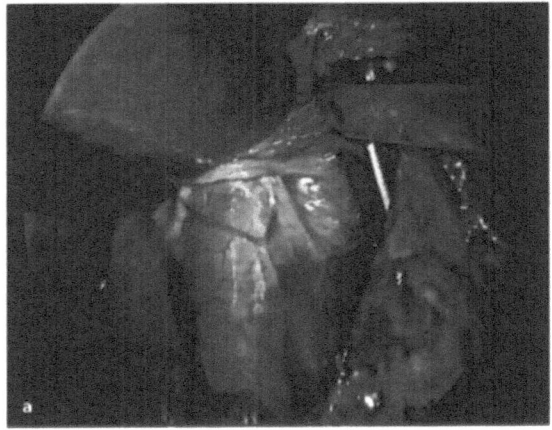

Fig. 2.7a. The left and right crus are identified and a window behind the esophagus is opened by blunt dissection (Hourlay Autostatic Retractor, Duchateau, Rouvreux, Belgium)

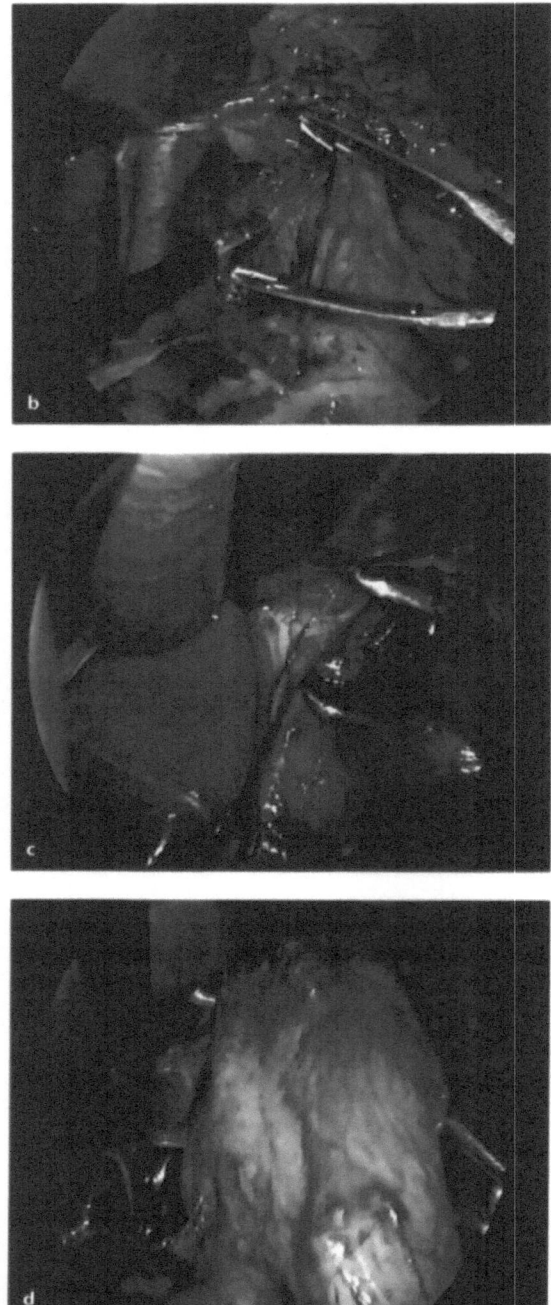

Fig. 2.7b–d

The whole procedure follows the principle of a "minimal paraesophageal dissection".

Using a roticular instrument (Roticulator Endograsp, AutoSuture, Norwalk, Conn. USA), the fundus is pulled through the window behind the esophagus (Fig. 2.8a,b).

The looseness of the wrap is given in our experience when the unfixed wrap stays in its position following the pull-through maneuver and does not slip back.

In case the wrap slips back, short gastric vessels are further divided and the dorsal plane of the fundus is again developed.

If this strategy again fails to give a loose wrap, we perform a dorsal hemifundoplication (Toupet).

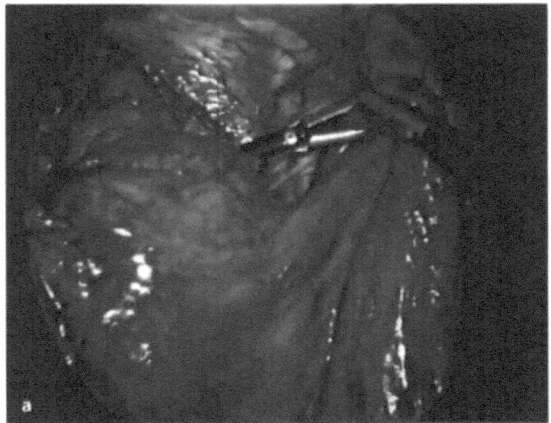

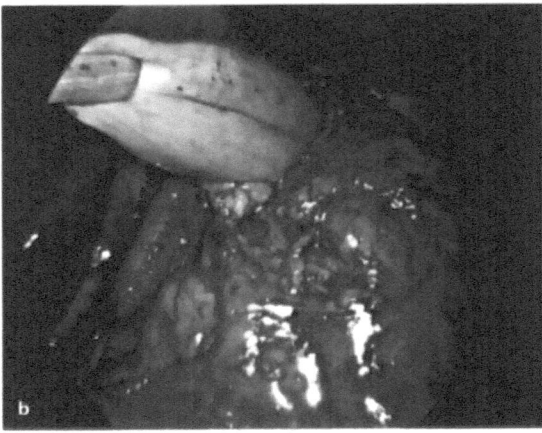

Fig. 2.8a,b. Using a roticular instrument, the fundus is pulled through the window behind the esophagus

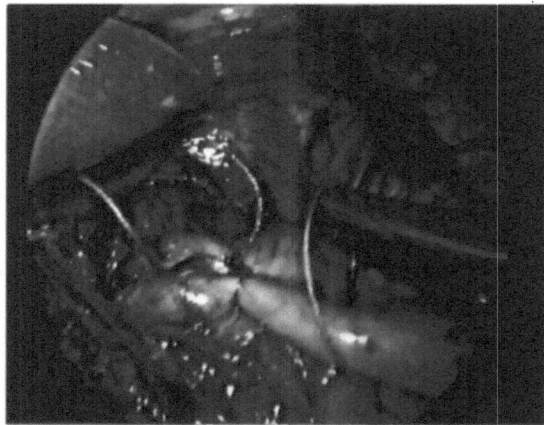

Fig. 2.9. Once fashioned, the wrap is fixed by two non-resorbable sutures knotted intracorporally over a distance of 2 cm

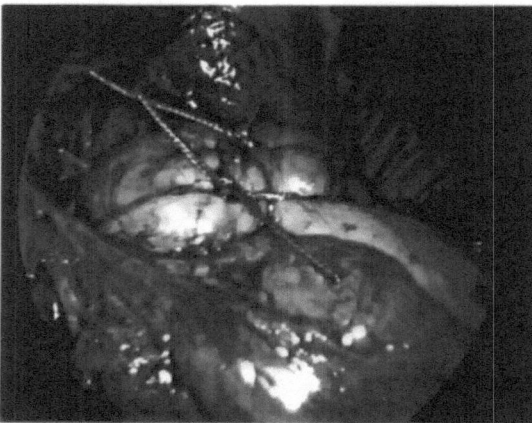

Fig. 2.10. The esophageal hiatus is repaired only when the bulk effect of the fundic wrap is considered to be insufficient to prevent herniation of intraperitoneal structures into the chest

Once the wrap is fashioned, it is fixed by two non-resorbable sutures (2–0 Ethibond) knot intracorporally (Fig. 2.9) over a distance of 2 cm.

The esophageal hiatus is repaired only when the bulk effect of the fundic wrap is considered to be insufficient to prevent herniation of intraperitoneal structures into the chest (Fig. 2.10).

Complications of Antireflux Surgery

1. *Perforation of the esophagus and stomach:* Perforation occurs in <1% of patients and is more common during the early learning curve and reoperation after failed antireflux surgery.
   In large paraesophageal hernias, it is advisable to pass a tube into the esophagus to see where to dissect in order to avoid the likelihood of esophageal injury. In some cases, gastroscopy may lead the way by diaphanoscopy more readily.
   Be aware that passing a tube from the esophagus into the stomach may cause perforation in paraesophageal hernias.
   Unrecognized perforation should be ruled out intraoperatively either by routinely performed gastroscopy or by inflating air via the gastric tube into the stomach. In the case of perforation, air bubbles are rising in the saline loaded upper abdominal region.

2. *Liver and spleen laceration:* Splenic injury is very uncommon in our experience, because the spleen lies dorsally to the primary dissecting plane. The left liver lobe is sometimes injured by the applied fan retractor. Bleeding can usually be controlled laparoscopically.

3. *Paraesophageal herniation:* The finding of a developing paraesophageal hernia a few days after fundoplication may be associated with the learning curve. The underlying mechanism may include technically inadequate crural repair. In our experience, forceful mobilization of a primarily short esophagus into the abdominal cavity and anchoring there by fundoplication and crural repair, moreover, may add a significant risk.

4. *Pneumothorax:* Particularly in large paraesophageal hernias, pneumothorax may occur by extensive mediastinal dissection of the esophagus and injury of the pleura.
   In intraoperative cardiopulmonary compromise, the possibility of a pneumothorax should promptly be taken into consideration and immediately reversed by inserting a chest tube.

5. *Dysphagia, "gas bloat" syndrome:* An excessively tight fundoplication results in dysphagia and the "gas bloat" syndrome (Fig. 2.11).
   By strictly applying the DeMeester modification of the original Nissen procedure (short, floppy, loose wrap), these complications have largely ceased to be a significant problem.

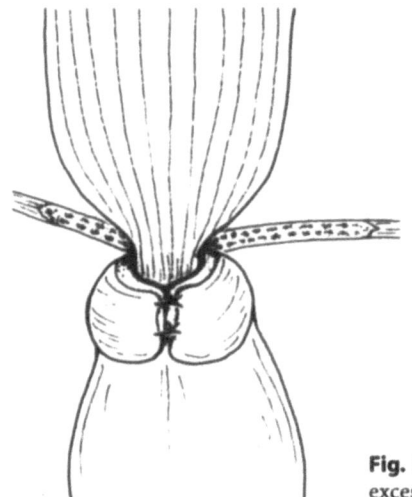

Fig. 2.11. Complications of antireflux surgery: excessively tight fundoplication results in dysphagia and the "gas bloat" syndrome

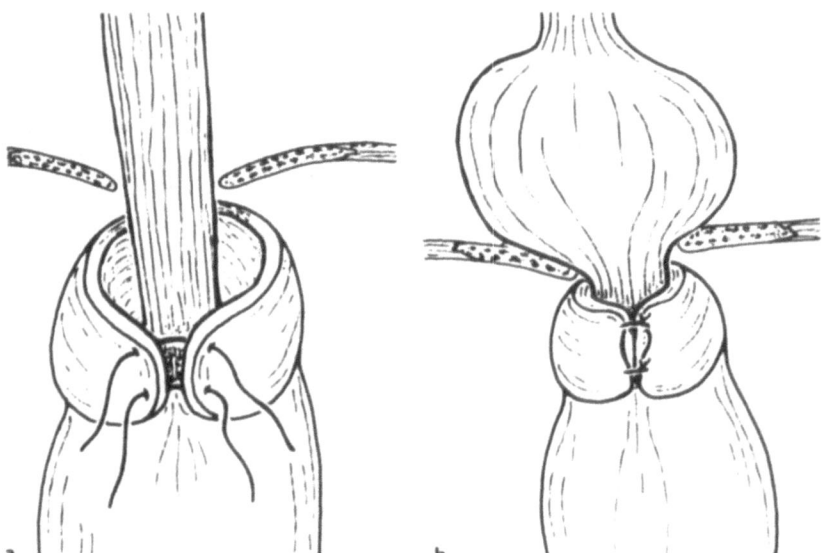

Fig. 2.12a,b. Complications of antireflux surgery: symptoms of recurrent reflux indicate disruption of the wrap or telescoping of the stomach through the wrap ("slipped" Nissen syndrome)

The surgeon should also be aware that even with medical therapy alone, many patients experience symptoms such as flatulence and bloating. If hypomotility of the tubular esophagus is present, even a correct short floppy wrap may result in dysphagia. Therefore, we recommend performing a partial fundoplication in these cases.

6. *Recurrent reflux:* Recurrent symptoms indicate disruption of the wrap or telescoping of the stomach through the wrap ("slipped" Nissen syndrome).(Fig. 2.12a,b).
Usually, the slipped wrap is attributed to inadequate fixation of the gastric wrap to the esophagus.
In our experience, the slipped wrap may be a true misnomer, because the wrap was incorrectly placed around the stomach rather than the esophagus.
Again, forceful mobilization of a primarily short elastic esophagus into the abdominal cavity may add a significant risk.

Overall Results of Laparoscopic Antireflux Surgery

All current reports on laparoscopic antireflux surgery suggest good symptomatic results with a low incidence of dysphagia and other side effects. Moreover, the reported morbidity and mortality is lower when compared to the open procedure.
Table 2.1 gives an overview of the worldwide experience with laparoscopic Nissen fundoplication.

Table 2.1. An overview of worldwide experience with laparoscopic Nissen fundoplication

Parameter	Number[a]	Percent
Mortality	4/2453	0.2
Conversion	143/2453	5.8
Early dysphagia	500/2453	20
Late dysphagia	114/2068	5.5
Dilatation/endoscopy	83/2068	4.0
Reoperation for dysphagia	18/2068	0.9
Recurrent reflux	57/1658	3.4
Reoperation for reflux	11/1658	0.7
Satisfaction	–	87 – 100

[a] Number of cases of total patients.

References

Anonymous (1997) Laparoscopic antireflux surgery for gastroesophageal reflux disease (GERD). Results of a Consensus Development Conference. Surg Endosc 11:413–426

Anonymous (1998) Guidelines for surgical treatment of gastroesophageal reflux disease (GERD). Surg Endosc 12:186–188

Anvari M, Allen Ch (1998) Laparoscopic Nissen fundoplication. Two-year comprehensive follow-up of a technique of minimal paraesophageal dissection. Ann Surg 227:25–32

Anvari M, Allen Ch, Borm A (1995) Laparoscopic Nissen fundoplication is a satisfactory alternative to long-term omeprazole therapy. Br J Surg 82:938–942

Crookes P, DeMeester T (1997) Complete and partial laparoscopic fundoplication for gastroesophageal reflux disease. Surg Endosc 11:613–614

Dallemagne B, Weerts J, Jehaes C, Markiewicz S, Lombard R (1991) Laparoscopic Nissen fundoplication: preliminary report. Surg Laparosc Endosc 3:138–143

Ferguson M (1997) Pitfalls and complications of antireflux surgery. Nissen and Collis-Nissen techniques. Chest Surg Clin North America 7:489–509

Fuchs KH, Freys SM, Heimbucher J, Thiede A (1993) Experiences with laparoscopic technique in anti-reflux surgery. Chirurg 64:317–23

Hinder R, Filipi Ch (1992) The technique of laparoscopic Nissen fundoplication. Surg Laparosc Endosc 3:265–272

Leggett P, Churchman-Winn R, Ahn C (1998) Resolving gastroesophageal reflux with laparoscopic fundoplication. Surg Endosc 12:142–147

Perdikis G, Hinder R, Lund R, Raiser F, Katada N (1997) Laparoscopic Nissen fundoplication: where do we stand? Surg Laparosc Endosc 7:17–21

Richardson W, Trus Th, Hunter J (1996) Laparoscopic antireflux surgery. Surg Clinics North America 76:437–450

Sampliner R (1998) Practice guidelines on the diagnosis, surveillance, and therapy of Barrett's esophagus. Am J Gastroenterol 93:1028–1032

Stein HJ, Feussner H, Siewet JR (1998) Indications for antireflux surgery of the oesophagus. Chirurg 69:132–40

Watson D, Jamieson G, Devitt P, Mitchell P, Game P (1995) Paraesophageal hiatus hernia: an important complication of laparoscopic Nissen fundoplication. Br J Surg 82:521–523

Achalasia: Pathophysiology, Diagnosis, and Nonoperative Treatment

T. Wehrmann and T. Schmitt

Pathophysiology

The first case description of a patient with a "megaesophagus" was in 1674 by Thomas Willis, but the term achalasia was first introduced into the medical literature by Sir Arthur Hurst in 1914. He not only recognized that failure of the lower esophageal sphincter to relax during deglutition is an important clinical feature of the disease, but also suggested that the lesion may be caused by a destruction of the normal esophageal neuroanatomy. Today, achalasia is a functional disorder characterized by almost complete disruption of the primary function of the esophagus; the transport of food from the pharynx to the stomach through the orderly process of peristalsis, which is synchronized with lower esophageal sphincter (LES) relaxation to allow entry into the stomach. Achalasia is a common cause of dysphagia, nocturnal regurgitation, and noncardiac chest pain (Achkar 1995; Anselmino et al. 1993; Shah et al. 1998; Dudnick et al. 1992).

Epidemiology

Achalasia affects males and females equally. It occurs in all races and does not predominate in white Caucasians alone. The high incidence in South America, especially in certain parts of Brazil, is due to Chagas' disease, an endemic disease caused by an infection with *Trypanosoma cruzi*. Otherwise, throughout the world, the incidence of patients diagnosed is approximately 1:100.000. Most patients in whom the diagnosis is made are between 35 and 45 years old. They have had their symptoms for about 5 years, although 20% have a 1-year history, and 20% longer than 10 years. In about 10%, the disease commenced in childhood. Neonates have been described, as well as have patients in their seventies. There is no evidence of any outbreaks suggesting an infective origin and there are no definite familial or hereditary influences in the few low-density epidemiological studies available, although a few siblings have been affected (Sugarbaker et al. 1993).

Pathology

The primary neurologic defect responsible for the development of achalasia remains unknown. Neuropathic changes have been noted at the LES, in the esophagus body, in the vagus nerves, and in the swallowing center of the central nervous system. The most consistent pathologic finding is at the LES, where an absence, decrease, or degeneration of ganglion cells in the myenteric plexus is usually seen. Occasionally, mild chronic inflammatory cell infiltration is seen around the remaining ganglion cells. Indirect evidence for the denervation of inhibitory nerves is seen in immunohistochemical studies of the LES. The inhibitory neuropeptide, vasoactive intestinal polypeptide (VIP), innervates the circular smooth muscle and myenteric plexus in normal patients. There is a marked decrease in VIP-containing nerve fibers in smooth muscle specimens from patients with achalasia as compared to control patients. Because VIP is a candidate neurotransmitter of physiologic LES relaxation, this reduced number of VIP-containing nerve fibers might account for the incomplete relaxation and increased resting pressure of the LES (Katada et al. 1996).

Abnormalities have also been found in the extrinsic neural pathway to the esophagus. Efferent parasympathetic innervation to the esophagus arises in the dorsal motor nucleus of the vagus. The cell bodies of this nucleus are distorted and reduced in number. Abnormalities of the vagus nerve trunks have also been reported. There, one may find degeneration of myelin sheaths and disintegration of axoplasm, suggestive of the wallerian degeneration seen after nerve transection. These findings suggest that in some patients, the primary defect is located in the preganglionic parasympathetic nerve supply to the esophagus (Perkin and Murray-Lyon 1998).

The smooth muscles of the esophagus and LES appear normal under light microscopy. Under electron microscopy, minor changes, such as detachment of the myofilaments from the surface membrane, alteration of cell size, and a paucity of intercellular junctions have been reported. These morphologic alterations in the esophageal smooth muscle cells are considered to result secondary to the denervation of the muscle (Milla 1996).

Pathophysiology

The smooth muscles of the gastrointestinal tract are under constant inhibitory tone. The elevated resting LES pressure may be caused by excitatory neural influences on the sphincter that are unopposed by inhibitory influences. Decreased inhibitory innervation could also explain the incomplete or absent sphincteric relaxation that occurs with swallowing. According to this hypothesis, the incomplete relaxation of the LES in achalasia is caused by the absence or functional impairment of the inhibitory innervation of the LES (Eckardt et al. 1995).

A genetic predisposition is supported by its occurrence among family members, a third of whom have consanguineous parents. Although most of these cases appear to be transmitted via a rare autosomal recessive trait, a single family has been reported in whom an autosomal dominant mode of inheritance with complete penetrance was observed. Further support for the importance of genetic factors comes from the observation that more than 80% of all patients with achalasia have the class II HLA, DQw1. Since class II antigens are frequently associated with autoimmune diseases, it could be speculated that a genetic predisposition exists that allows destruction of neural cells by an autoimmune process that is perhaps initiated by viral infections (Koshy and Nostrant 1997; De la Concha et al. 1998).

Physiologic abnormalities in achalasia supporting the presence of lower esophageal sphincter denervation include the following:
1. Basal hypertonicity
2. Incomplete relaxation
3. The presence of hypersensitivity to cholinergic agonists and gastrin
4. Excitatory responses of the LES to cholecystokinin.

Diagnosis

Clinical Presentation

Patients with achalasia typically suffer from symptoms for several years before the final diagnosis is made. In a study carried out in Germany by Eckardt et al. (1997a), the mean duration of symptoms at the time of diagnosis was 4.7 years and most of the 87 patients had consulted at least two physicians before the correct diagnosis was made. This was mainly due to a misinterpretation of the patients' symptoms by their primary physicians and not caused by atypical clinical presentation (Birgisson and Richter 1997; Meshkinpour et al. 1994).

The cardinal symptoms of achalasia are dysphagia, regurgitation and pulmonary aspiration, weight loss, and chest discomfort. The most striking feature of achalasia is dysphagia for both solids and liquids, which is usually moderately progressive, often resulting in a significant weight loss over several months or years. A very rapid loss of weight (< 3 months) is not typical of achalasia, but is often observed in patients with malignant esophageal obstruction. The main differential diagnoses include reflux disease, benign or malignant esophageal stenosis, scleroderma, or other esophageal motility disorders such as diffuse esophageal spasm. In addition, patients with bulimia or anorexia nervosa may sometimes be incorrectly diagnosed as suffering from achalasia because they induce regurgitation after meals to reduce chest pain or avoid ingestion of solid foods.

Endoscopy

The first investigation generally performed in patients with dysphagia is upper gastrointestinal (GI) endoscopy. Thereby, some differential diagnoses to achalasia, such as benign or malignant esophageal stenosis, reflux esophagitis, or large diverticula, can be ruled out. After passing the cardia with the endoscope, careful inspection of the gastroesophageal junction should be made on retroflex view (Figs. 3.1, 3.2, see also Fig. 3.5). In particular, secondary achalasia due to carcinoma of the gastric cardia (Fig. 3.2) must be excluded (Streitz et al. 1995).

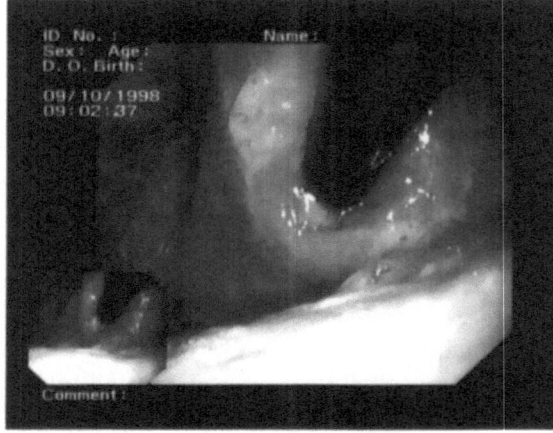

Fig. 3.1. Normal endoscopic view (retroflexed instrument) of the gastric cardia

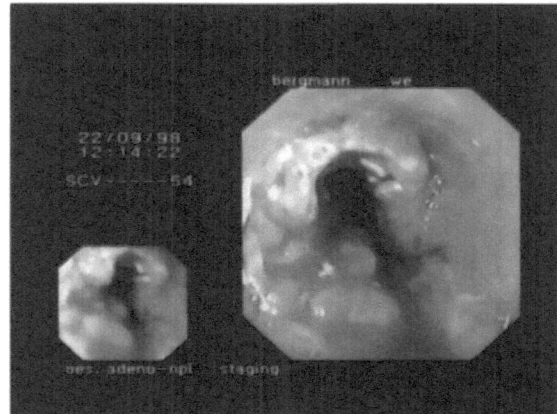

Fig. 3.2. Adenocarcinoma of the gastric cardia on endocospic view

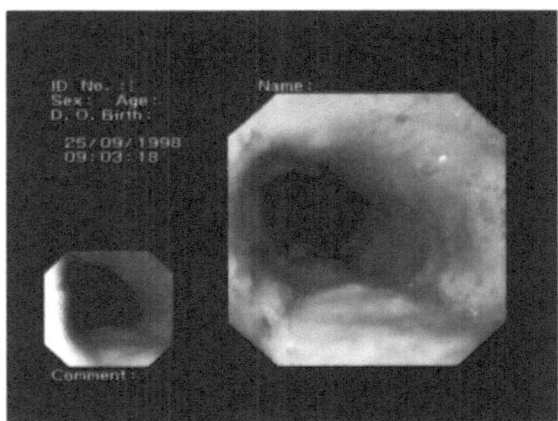

Fig. 3.3. Dilated esophageal body (endoscopic appearance) with food retention in an achalasia patient

In patients with achalasia, it may sometimes be necessary to lavage the esophagus by means of a nasogastric tube before endoscopic inspection due to esophageal retention of solid foods (Fig. 3.3). Typical endoscopic findings of achalasia include dilatation and absence of peristaltic activity of the esophageal body with normal mucosa (Fig. 3.3). However, erosive esophagitis may also be present due to retention of debris and food.

The cardia usually has a puckered appearance that does not open with air insufflation (Fig. 3.4). However, the endoscope should easily traverse the cardia into the gastric fundus by the application of only gentle forward pressure on the instrument. Inability to pass the endoscope through the gastroesophageal junction, or the necessity for undue force

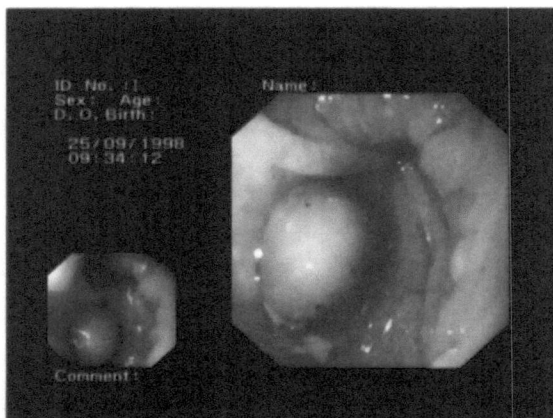

Fig. 3.4. Puckered appearance of the cardia at prograde endoscopic view in an achalasia patient (with esophageal food retention)

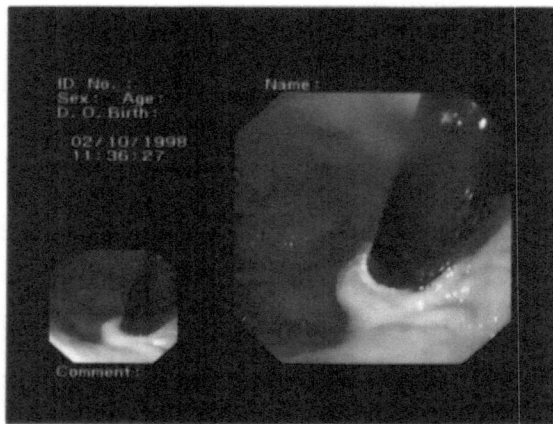

Fig. 3.5. Hypercompetent lower esophageal sphincter in achalasia (endoscopic, retroflexed view)

during this maneuver, should raise the suspicion of malignancy or a benign stricture of the cardia. In such cases, retroflex inspection and endosonographic examination of the cardia must be carried out by bougienage. In primary achalasia, the retroflex view of the cardia often impressively revealed the hypercompetent LES (Fig. 3.5).

An interesting technique that can be used to further evaluate the LES endoscopically in this situation is measurement of the intragastric pressure (via the working channel of the endoscope) required to force open the sphincter (so-called yield pressure). Air is pumped into the stomach until the cardia is seen to open and an audible belch is heard (McGouran et al. 1988). Normal subjects were found to have a yield pressure of up to 9 mmHg, whereas patients with achalasia revealed a mean yield pressure of 21 mmHg. Furthermore, a recent study demonstrated that by careful videoendoscopic observation of (dry) swallow-induced esophageal peristalsis and the ability of the cardia to open during swallowing, a correct diagnosis of achalasia can be made in 96% of cases by endoscopy alone (Cameron et al. 1999).

Radiology

Achalasia can be suspected from unusual findings on plain chest X-rays, e.g., an air–fluid level indicative of retained esophageal secretions, displacement of the trachea by a dilated esophagus, or the lack of gastric air collection. Pulmonary infiltrates may result from chronic aspiration in patients with long-standing achalasia.

The barium swallow under fluoroscopy has always been the primary method of motor function evaluation in achalasia. It has the clear advantage vs. esophageal manometry (see below) to be easily available and well tolerated (Chawda et al. 1998; Mirchandani et al. 1995).

During continuous fluoroscopic monitoring, it is clearly seen that the peristalsis fails to clear the esophagus after barium ingestion. Contrast material may simply lie in the atonic esophagus or be moved up and

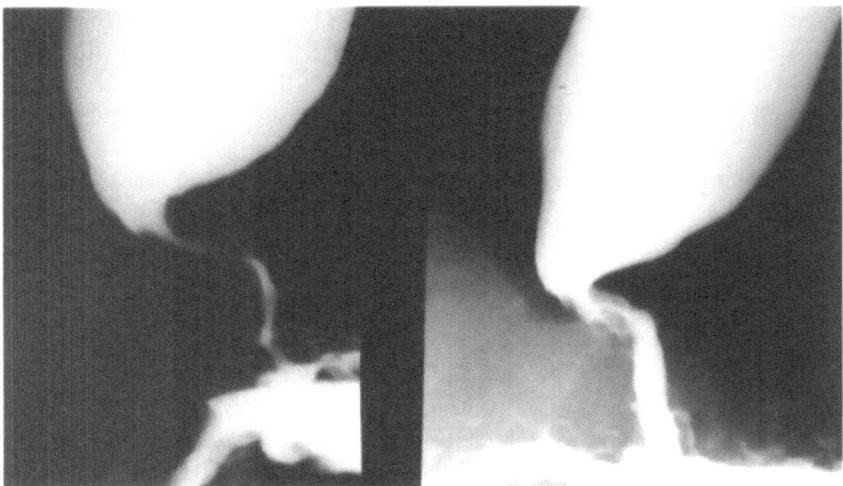

Fig. 3.6. Dilated esophagus and "bird-beak" appearance of the gastric cardia in achalasia (barium swallow). Radiographic appearance before (*left*) and 2 months after botulinum toxin injection (*right*)

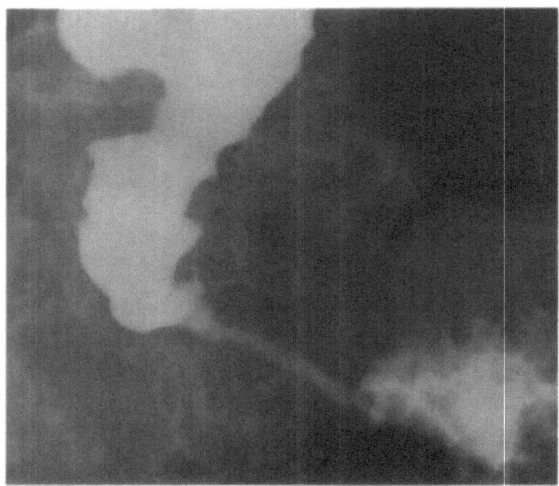

Fig. 3.7. Epiphrenic diverticulum in a patient with long-standing achalasia

down the esophageal body by repetitive, non-peristaltic contractions (so-called tertiary contractions). The gastric cardia opens partially and intermittently, allowing only small amounts of contrast material to pass into the fundus.

After complete barium filling of the esophagus, marked dilatation of the esophageal body often becomes evident (Fig. 3.6). The dilatation is greatest in the distal part of the esophagus. In the early stage of achalasia, or in some patients with vigorous achalasia, esophageal dilatation may be absent. In long-standing disease, the dilatation may distort the normal esophageal anatomy, making it resemble a sigmoid colon, also called a "tortuous megaesophagus".

The column of barium terminates in a tapered point, the non-relaxing LES. This finding is commonly known as the "birds beak" (Fig. 3.6). Occasionally, an epiphrenic diverticulum is associated with achalasia (Falk 1994) (Fig. 3.7).

Esophageal Manometry

Still today, esophageal manometry remains the gold standard for establishing the diagnosis of achalasia. Manometry is particularly recommended in patients with atypical symptoms or only discrete pathology on barium X-ray. On the other hand, for clinical purposes, patients with typical presentation and obvious radiographic findings did not need esophageal manometry (Freidin et al. 1992).

Table 3.1. Manometric features of achalasia

Parameter	Normal	Achalasia
LES relaxation	>60%	≤60%
LES resting pressure[a]	10–35 mmHg	>35 mmHg
Proportion of simultaneous contractions (distal esophageal body)	≤10%	>10%
Contraction amplitude[a] (distal esophageal body)	40–160 mmHg	<40 mmHg

LES, lower esophageal sphincter. [a]Facultative findings.

Esophageal manometry can be performed with either water-perfused catheters or with solid state transducers. Before the manometry catheter is inserted, the esophagus should be cleaned of retained particles of solid food. It is occasionally difficult to advance the manometry probe through the gastric cardia, but perseverance is important as LES relaxation must be evaluated. Fluoroscopic guidance and the use of a (formerly placed endoscopically) guidewire-armed manometry probe may help with placement. The characteristic manometric features of achalasia are given by Table 3.1. The absence of peristaltic activity in the esophageal body after swallowing of liquids and reduced swallow-induced relaxation of the LES are prerequisites for the diagnosis. The contraction waves are usually of low amplitude (<40 mmHg) and are simultaneous in onset (Fig. 3.8). Some patients may exhibit higher amplitude (>80 mmHg), simultaneous repetitive contractions in response to swallowing, known as vigorous achalasia (for details see above). The question of whether this is a real, distinct clinical entity remains unclear.

In about two thirds of patients, the LES resting pressure is elevated (>35 mmHg) (Fig. 3.8). Very low sphincter pressures (<5–10 mmHg) are not seen in achalasia and should suggest another diagnosis, such as scleroderma or severe reflux disease. More important for the diagnosis of achalasia than the LES resting pressure is the demonstration of impaired LES relaxation after swallowing (Fig. 3.8). In nearly all patients, sphincter relaxation of less than 60% can be documented by manometry after swallowing of a 5-ml water bolus.

Several other disorders can mimic the manometric findings of achalasia. In secondary achalasia due to mechanical compression of the cardia by adenocarcinoma or physical disruption of the myenteric plexus by neoplastic infiltration (mainly by lymphomas), LES relaxation may be completely absent. Furthermore, infection with Trypanosoma cruzi results in the destruction of ganglia of the myenteric plexus and produc-

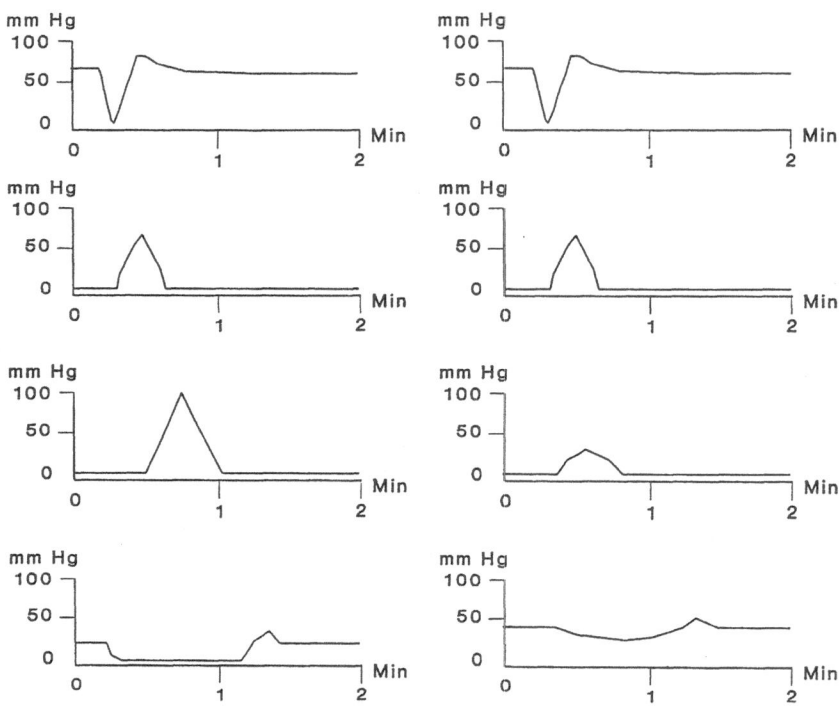

Fig. 3.8. Esophageal manometry in health (*left*) and achalasia (*right*)

tion of an esophageal syndrome similar to achalasia. The so-called Chagas' disease is endemic in South America (particularly in Brazil). Unlike achalasia, clinical involvement of the small intestine and the colon, as well as the heart and urinary tract, is common in patients with Chagas' disease. Very seldom, amyloidosis of the esophagus produces an achalasia-like picture (aperistalsis and impairment of LES relaxation).

Nonoperative Treatment

None of the currently available therapeutic modalities will correct the underlying neural defects of achalasia. Therefore, the main goal of therapy is to improve esophageal emptying and to give relief from dysphagia. The first treatment option described was esophageal bougienage with a whale bone by Sir Thomas Willis in 1674. However, symptomatic improvement following simple bougienage is brief because longer lasting improvement can only be achieved by significant disruption of LES muscle fibers. By this mechanism, the obstructing LES may be overcome by improved gravitational esophageal emptying as a consequence of the reduced LES tone. The abnormal LES relaxation, however, could not be corrected by any form of treatment (Saigal and Kumar 1996). Significant disruption of the LES fibers can be achieved by pneumatic dilatation and by operative cardiomyotomy. Nowadays, both these methods are the most common and successful forms of treatment. Most patients (>80%) benefited from both treatment modalities, although one study (Meshkinpour et al. 1994) showed that about half of the successfully treated patients reported residual symptoms which had an impact on their lifestyle. Only just recently, endoscopic botulinum toxin (BTX) injection has been introduced as a minimally invasive technique for the treatment of achalasia patients (Albanese et al. 1995; Allescher and Ravich 1993; Annese et al. 1998; Bhutani 1997; Hoffman et al. 1997; Pasricha et al. 1994).

Medical Treatment

Up to now, no pharmacological agent has been proven to give sustained long-term improvement. A number of drugs (e.g., anticholinergics, amyl nitrate, nitroglycerin, theophylline, and b-agonists) act on the LES smooth muscle directly or indirectly to reduce the resting sphincter tone in healthy volunteers and patients with achalasia (Bortolotti 1999; Bortolotti et al. 1994; Pasricha and Kalloo 1997; Walker 1997).

The greatest experience exists with nitrates and calcium channel blockers (e.g., isorbide dinitrate 10 mg t.i.d. or nifedipine 10–20 mg t.i.d.). By directly relaxing smooth muscle, these compounds decrease LES pressure and may reduce the vigor of non-peristaltic contractions in the esophageal body. Increased esophageal radionuclide emptying and improvement of symptoms have been documented in several studies. However, results from other groups found only minimal clinical benefit from medical therapy. The efficacy of long-term use of nitrates and calcium antagonists has not been documented, but symptom control has been observed for at least 1.5 years. Side effects (especially headache) are commonly observed under medical treatment. Therefore, the exact role of pharmacological agents in the management of achalasia remains unclear. In our opinion, pharmacotherapy for achalasia should be reserved for those candidates who have mild symptoms or wish to delay definite therapy.

Pneumatic Dilatation

Since the effect of bougienage is usually transient, pneumatic dilatation has replaced bougienage as the first-line treatment of patients with achalasia (Schwartz et al. 1993). For this procedure, devices with expanding metal arms (Starck) and nylon or latex balloons of varying diameter (2–5 cm), expanded either by air or water pressure (i.e., those developed by Mosher, Walter Palmer, Hurst–Tucker, Brown–McHardy, Rider–Moeller, and other devices), were used. In the late 1980s, the Rigiflex dilator (Microvasive, Watertown, USA) was developed with a double-lumen catheter allowing placement of the entire dilator over a guidewire (Fig. 3.9). The cylindrical balloon is made of non-radiopaque polyethylene and available in three diameters (3, 3.5, and 4 cm). Another type of dilator (Witzel) is a non-radiopaque polyethylene balloon mounted on a forward-viewing endoscope, making it possible to position and inflate the balloon device under direct (retroflexed) endoscopic vision. Today, the Rigiflex system, in particular, has gained widespread use. However, the technique of pneumatic dilatation for achalasia is far from standardized. Not only balloon type and size, but also premedication and balloon inflation pressure and duration vary between centers.

We have been employing the following technique for the last 10 years using the Rigiflex balloon dilator: After a liquid diet for 24 h and overnight fasting, the patient's esophagus was cleaned from residual food and debris by means of a 24-gauge nasogastric tube. Thereafter, the patient received pre-medication of either 5 mg of midazolam, or repeti-

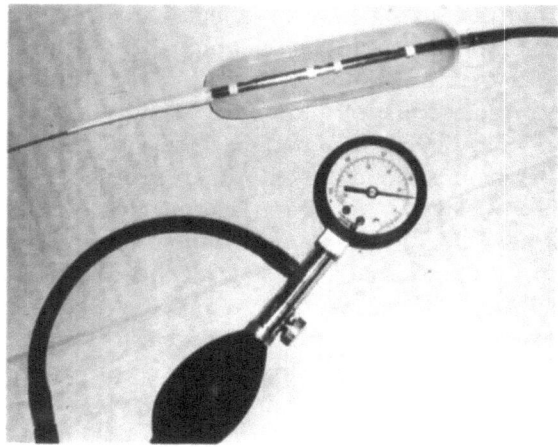

Fig. 3.9. Rigiflex dilator with guidewire for treatment of achalasia

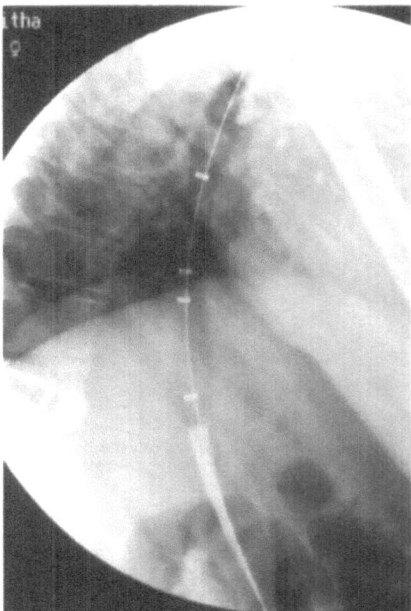 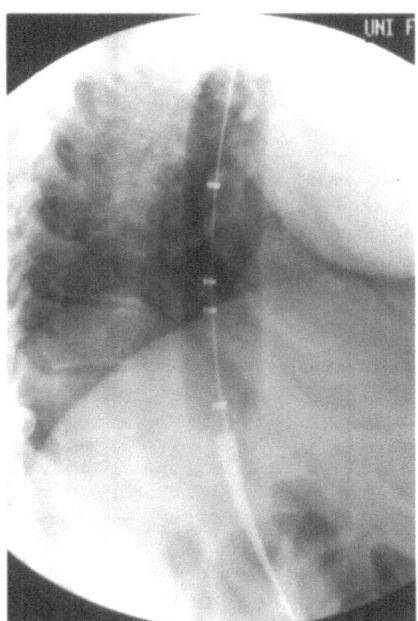

Fig. 3.10. Placed Rigiflex dilator at the gastric cardia

Fig. 3.11. Inflated Rigiflex dilator

tive doses of propofol intravenously. After endoscopic insertion of an Eder–Puestow guidewire into the stomach, the polyethylene Rigiflex balloon device is introduced and placed under fluoroscopic control in the esophagogastric junction (Fig. 3.10). Two different balloon sizes (30 or 35 mm) were used, depending on the maximal diameter (obtained from a barium swallow) of the narrowed cardia segment (30-mm balloon if the diameter was smaller than or equal to 3 mm at radiology and 35-mm balloon if the diameter exceeded 3 mm, respectively). If the patient underwent a repeated dilatation procedure, this was always performed with the 35-mm balloon.

After correct placement of the device, rapid inflation of the balloon with air is performed (Fig. 3.11). Balloon pressure is continuously monitored throughout the whole procedure and kept constant at 7 psi, at which complete obliteration of the balloon waist can be observed during the procedure. The first inflation is held for 2 min, and after a 2-min rest, a second inflation over 3 min is performed with identical pressure.

After the dilatation procedure, the patient is checked for possible esophageal perforation by repeated endoscopic examination and, in the

Table 3.2. Results and complications of pneumatic dilatation in the treatment of achalasia

Reference	Dilatation device	Number	Symptomatic relief (%)	Perforation incidence (%)
Csendes (1991)	Mosher	39	65	5
Stark (1990)	Brown – McHardy	10	100	0
Eckardt et al. (1992)	Brown – McHardy	54	78	2
Parkmann (1993)	Brown – McHardy	123	88	2
Coccia (1991)	Rider – Moeller	16	75	0
Bourgeois (1991)	Rider – Moeller	53	80	4
Gelfand (1989)	Rigiflex	24	83	0
Stark (1990)	Rigiflex	10	70	0
Nadakia (1995)	Rigiflex	29	93	0
Wehrmann (1995)	Rigiflex	40	88	3
Vaezi et al. (1999)	Rigiflex	20	75	5

case of any doubts, by means of a 20-ml swallow of water-soluble contrast medium under X-ray monitoring. Thereafter, the patient is kept in hospital overnight.

By using different balloon devices and dilatation techniques, short-term symptomatic improvement can be expected in nearly 70% – 90% of achalasia patients (Bernstein and Barkin 1993; Bhatnagar et al. 1996; Fiest et al. 1993; Kozarek et al. 1995; Matsuo et al. 1992; Molina et al. 1996; Ponce et al. 1996). The current data from the literature are summarized in Table 3.2.

It has been demonstrated that patients who are older (> 45 years) and in whom a reduction of the LES resting pressure below 15 mmHg could be achieved will have a more favorable outcome (Eckardt et al. 1992; Wehrmann et al. 1995).

Esophageal perforation is the most common and hazardous complication of pneumatic dilatation, but (sub-)mucosal hematoma, hemorrhage, fever, or a sterile pleural effusion may also occur. The incidence of perforation is quoted at about 3% in the literature (Table 3.2). In the case of perforation, the patient rarely requires surgical intervention (only if a bright mediastinal rupture is obvious or a pleural involvement is noted), but in most instances can be managed conseratively by immediate endoscopic placement of a 6-F nasomediastinal tube (for drainage of potentially bacterial contaminated esophagogastric juice in the mediastinal perforation site), parenteral nutrition, and medication with i.v. broad-spectrum antibiotics and proton-pump inhibitors. The mucosal perforation site can be closed endoscopically some days later by fibrin glue or by means of hemoclip application.

By 24 h, intraesophageal pH-metry prolonged acid exposure could be documented after pneumatic dilatation, but clinically important gastro-esophageal reflux disease rarely occurred (Wehrmann et al. 1995; Shoe-nut et al. 1997).

Regarding long-term efficacy of pneumatic dilatation, only sparse data are available. Nearly one third of the patients developed symptom recurrence during the 10 years following pneumatic dilatation. Efficacy of pneumatic dilatation is reduced by half for each subsequent proce-dure and, therefore, approximately 10% of the patients who initially had been treated with forceful dilatation, later had to undergo operative car-diomyotomy (Gupta et al. 1997; Kalicinski et al. 1997; Kumar et al. 1994; Livingstone and Sosa 1995; Malthaner et al. 1994; Mbembati et al. 1994; Parrilla et al. 1992; Pricolo et al. 1993). Results of cardiomyotomy are not influenced by previous dilatation. There is only one study group which prospectively compared the results of pneumatic dilatation and that of operative cardiomyotomy (Csendes et al. 1991). The authors found that surgery gave better long-term improvement than forceful dilatation. Because the efficacy of pneumatic dilatation in these series seemed less than in other trials, this conclusion has been questioned.

Botulinum Toxin Injection

Botulinum toxin A is a neurotoxin from *Clostridium botulinum* that inhibits the release of acetylcholine from cholinergic nerve endings (Schiano et al. 1998). The toxin has been used since 1980 to provide relief for a variety of skeletal muscle spastic disorders, such as strabismus, tor-ticollis spasticus, and hemifacial spasm. The use of the drug in these dis-orders has been limited by the need for repeated injections every few months (since the effects of BTX wane over time), and an observed

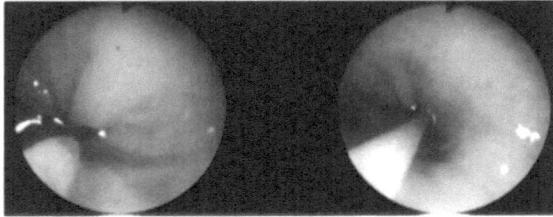

Fig. 3.12. Endoscopic botulinum toxin injection at the lower esophageal sphincter (endoscopic view)

declining effectiveness of repeated injections due to an unclear mechanism (development of blocking antibodies, etc.). Pasricha and coworkers (1995) from Baltimore were the first to apply local injection of BTX into the LES in patients with achalasia (Fig. 3.12). Formerly, they had been shown that intrasphincteric BTX injection significantly reduced the LES tone in piglets (Pasricha et al. 1994). This approach was shown to lead to short-term (4–8 weeks) symptom relief in up to 90% of patients (Table 3.3, Fig. 3.13).

By 6 months, 20 of 31 (65%) achalasia patients treated with intrasphincteric injection of 80 U of BTX by the group from Pasricha et al. (1996) were still in clinical remission, with a mean remission period of 15 months (range, 5–29 months). However, several other trials could not confirm these initial results (Table 3.3). For example, in our own study (Wehrmann et al. 1999), we found a mean remission period of only 5 months (range, 2–9 months).

Fishman et al. (1996) demonstrated that re-iterative BTX injection is not effective if the initial BTX administration is ineffective (BTX nonresponder). However, there is some evidence that there is a trend towards a longer lasting symptomatic response after repeated BTX injections than after the initial treatment of primary BTX responders.

The endoscopic BTX injection procedure is simple, can be done on an outpatient basis, and no major complications have been reported as yet. When comparing BTX injection with pneumatic dilatation, Annese et al.

Table 3.3. Results of botulinum toxin (BTX) injection in achalasia

Reference	Number	BTX dose	Initial success (%)	Number of re-injections	Long-term response (%)	Follow-up (months)
Pasricha et al. (1996)	31	80	90	1.6	68	12
Fishman et al. (1996)	60	80	70	1.3	36	12
Cuilliere et al. (1997)	55	80	85	1.2	60	6
Gordon and Eaker (1997)	16	80	75	1.25	58	7
Wehrmann et al. 1999	20	100	80	2.5	70	24
Vaezi et al. 1999	22	100	64	1.1	32	12

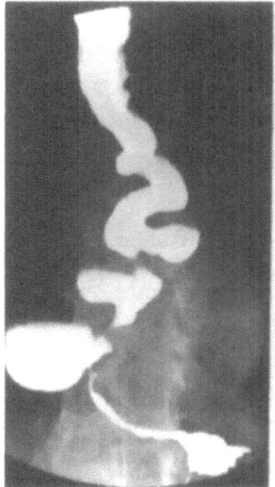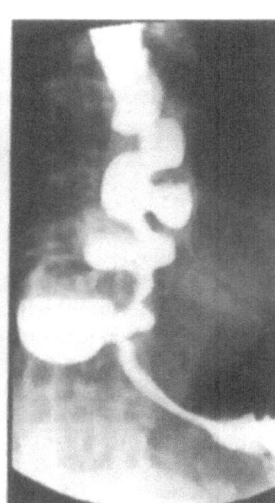

Fig. 3.13 Same patient as in Fig. 3.7, before (*left*) and 2 months after botulinum toxin injection (barium swallow)

(1996b) showed similar results for both treatment forms after 12 months of follow-up in a small cohort of patients. Their study designed to dilate only patients who initially did not respond to BTX, however, renders the comparison unfair. In a recent study by Vaezi and colleagues (1999), 14 of 20 (70%) patients after pneumatic dilatation compared with only seven of 22 (32%) patients after BTX injection were still in clinical remission at 12 months. Moreover, BTX injection, in contrast to pneumatic dilatation, did not have a significant effect on objective parameters such as LES pressure or radiographic findings, even at 1 month after intervention. However, these results were obtained by performing a single injection of BTX only. Other studies, like our own (Wehrmann et al. 1999), have shown that about 70% of achalasia patients could be satisfactorily managed by repeated (median, three) BTX injections during long-term follow-up (1–4 years).

Up to now, it is not well defined which achalasia patients are the best candidates for BTX treatment. In our opinion, these are patients with local (tortuous megaesophagus and/or epiphrenic diverticulum) or systemic (advanced age and/or serious co-morbidity) risk factors, rendering dilatation and cardiomyotomy very risky. It may also be an alternative for patients wishing to delay definite therapy.

In today's era of patient awareness and self-determination, the physician must discuss the pros and cons of cardiomyotomy, pneumatic dilatation, and BTX injection with the achalasia patient (Topart et al. 1992;

Vaezi and Richter 1998; Yoneyama et al. 1998). Thereafter, the patient may choose one therapy over another on the basis of objective information, but also with regard to personal fears, beliefs, and preferences.

References

Achkar E (1995) Achalasia. Gastroenterologist 3:273 – 288

Albanese A, Bentivoglio AR, Cassetta E et al. (1995) Review article: the use of botulinum toxin in the alimentary tract. Aliment Pharmacol Ther 9:599 – 604

Allescher HD, Ravich WJ (1993) Medical treatment of esophageal motility disorders. Dysphagia 8:125 – 134

Annese V, Basciani M, Lombardi G et al. (1996a) Perendoscopic injection of botulinum toxin is effective in achalasia after failure of myotomy or pneumatic dilation. Gastrointest Endosc 44:461 – 465

Annese V, Basciani M, Perri F et al. (1996b) Controlled trial of botulinum toxin injection versus placebo and pneumatic dilation in achalasia. Gastroenterology 111:1418 – 1424

Annese V, Basciani M, Borrelli O et al. (1998) Intrasphincteric injection of botulinum toxin is effective in long-term treatment of esophageal achalasia. Muscle Nerve 21:1540 – 1542

Anselmino M, Clark GW, Hinder RA (1993) Esophageal chest pain: state of the art. Surg Annu 25:193 – 210

Bernstein D, Barkin JS (1993) Pneumatic dilation of a sigmoid esophagus in achalasia using an overtube. Gastrointest Endosc 39:549 – 550

Bhatnagar MS, Nanivadekar SA, Sawant P et al. (1996) Achalasia cardia dilatation using polyethylene balloon (Rigiflex) dilators. Indian J Gastroenterol 15:49 – 51

Bhutani MS (1997) Gastrointestinal uses of botulinum toxin. Am J Gastroenterol 92:929 – 933

Birgisson S, Richter JE (1997) Achalasia: what's new in diagnosis and treatment? Dig Dis 15:1 – 27

Bortolotti M (1999) Medical therapy of achalasia: a benefit reserved for few. Digestion 60:11 – 16

Bortolotti M, Coccia G, Brunelli F et al. (1994) Isosorbide dinitrate or nifedipine: which is preferable in the medical therapy of achalasia? Ital J Gastroenterol 26:379 – 382

Cameron AJ, Malcolm A, Prather CM et al. (1999) Videoendoscopic diagnosis of esophageal motility disorders. Gastrointest Endosc 49:62 – 69

Chawda SJ, Watura R, Adams H et al. (1998) A comparison of barium swallow and erect esophageal transit scintigraphy following balloon dilatation for achalasia. Dis Esophagus 11:181 – 187 (discussion 187 – 188)

Csendes A (1991) Results of surgical treatment of achalasia of the esophagus. Hepatogastroenterology 38:474 – 480

Cuilliere C, Ducrotte P, Zerbib F et al. (1997) Achalasia: outcome of patients treated with intrasphincteric injection of botulinum toxin. Gut 41:87 – 92

De la Concha EG, Fernandez-Arquero M, Mendoza JL et al. (1998) Contribution of HLA class II genes to susceptibility in achalasia. Tissue Antigens 52:381 – 384

Dudnick RS, Castell JA, Castell DO (1992) Abnormal upper esophageal sphincter function in achalasia. Am J Gastroenterol 87:1712–1715

Eckardt VF, Aignherr C, Bernhard G (1992) Predictors of outcome in patients with achalasia treated by pneumatic dilation. Gastroenterology 103:1732–1738

Eckardt VF, Stenner F, Liewen H et al. (1995) Autonomic dysfunction in patients with achalasia. Neurogastroenterol Motil 7:55–61

Eckardt VF, Kanzler G, Westermeier T (1997a) Complications and their impact after pneumatic dilation for achalasia: prospective long-term follow-up study. Gastrointest Endosc 45:349–353

Eckardt VF, Kohne U, Junginger T et al. (1997b) Risk factors for diagnostic delay in achalasia. Dig Dis Sci 42:580–585

Falk GW (1994) Regurgitation in a patient with an esophageal diverticulum. Cleve Clin J Med 61:409–411

Fiest TC, Foong A, Chokhavatia S (1993) Successful balloon dilation of achalasia during pregnancy. Gastrointest Endosc 39:810–812

Fishman VM, Parkman HP, Schiano TD et al. (1996) Symptomatic improvement in achalasia after botulinum toxin injection of the lower esophageal sphincter. Am J Gastroenterol 91:1724–1730

Freidin N, Eidelman S, Danieli Z et al. (1992) Insertion of Dent sleeve catheter using a guidewire in achalasia. Gastrointest Endosc 38:699–700

Gordon JM, Eaker EY (1997) Prospective study of esophageal botulinum toxin injection in high-risk achalasia patients. Am J Gastroenterol 92:1812–1817

Gupta NM, Goenka MK, Behera A et al. (1997) Transhiatal oesophagectomy for benign obstructive conditions of the oesophagus. Br J Surg 84:262–264

Hoffman BJ, Knapple WL, Bhutani MS et al. (1997) Treatment of achalasia by injection of botulinum toxin under endoscopic ultrasound guidance. Gastrointest Endosc 45:77–79

Kadakia SC (1993) Coping with achalasia. Postgrad Med 93:249–250, 253–258, 260

Kalicinski P, Dluski E, Drewniak T et al. (1997) Esophageal manometric studies in children with achalasia before and after operative treatment. Pediatr Surg Int 12:571–575

Katada N, Hinder RA, Hinder PR et al. (1996) The hypertensive lower esophageal sphincter. Am J Surg 172:439–442 (discussion 442–443)

Koshy SS, Nostrant TT (1997) Pathophysiology and endoscopic/balloon treatment of esophageal motility disorders. Surg Clin North Am 77:971–992

Kozarek RA, Patterson DJ, Ball TJ et al. (1995) Esophageal dilation can be done safely using selective fluoroscopy and single dilating sessions. J Clin Gastroenterol 20:184–188

Kumar A, Wig JD, Kochhar R et al. (1994) An audit of pneumatic dilatation and oesophagomyotomy in patients with achalasia cardia. Trop Gastroenterol 15:152–156

Livingstone AS, Sosa JL (1995) Surgical laparoscopy: impact on the management of abdominal disorders. Dig Dis 13:56–67

Malthaner RA, Tood TR, Miller L et al. (1994) Long-term results in surgically managed esophageal achalasia. Ann Thorac Surg 58:1343–1346 (discussion 1346–1347)

Matsuo Y, Sugimura F, Seki A (1992) Long-term prognosis of patients with achalasia treated by cardial dilatation therapy. Gastroenterol Jpn 27:719–727

Mbembati NA, Lema LE, Kahamba JF et al. (1994) Operative management of achalasia of the oesophagus. East Afr Med J 71:421–423

McGouran RC, Galloway JM, Spence DS et al. (1988) Does measurement of yield pressure at the cardia during endoscopy provide information on the function of the lower oesophageal sphincter mechanism? Gut 29:275–278

Meshkinpour H, Haghighat P, Dutton C (1994) Clinical spectrum of esophageal aperistalsis in the elderly. Am J Gastroenterol 89:1480–1483

Milla PJ (1996) Intestinal motility during ontogeny and intestinal pseudo-obstruction in children. Pediatr Clin North Am 43:511–532

Mirchandani LV, Joshi JM (1995) Achalasia cardia – perplexing chest radiographs. J Assoc Physicians India 43:721–722

Molina EG, Stollman N, Grauer L et al. (1996) Conservative management of esophageal nontransmural tears after pneumatic dilation for achalasia. Am J Gastroenterol 91:15–18

Parrilla P, Aguayo JL, Martinez de Haro L et al. (1992) Reversible achalasia-like motor pattern of esophageal body secondary to postoperative stricture of gastroesophageal junction. Dig Dis Sci 37:1781–1784

Pasricha PJ, Kalloo AN (1997) Recent advances in the treatment of achalasia. Gastrointest Endosc Clin N Am 7:191–206

Pasricha PJ, Ravich WJ, Hendrix TR et al. (1994) Treatment of achalasia with intrasphincteric injection of botulinum toxin. A pilot trial. Ann Intern Med 121:590–591

Pasricha PJ, Ravich WJ, Hendrix TR et al. (1995) Intrasphincteric botulinum toxin for the treatment of achalasia. N Engl J Med 332:774–778

Pasricha PJ, Rai R, Ravich WJ et al. (1996) Botulinum toxin for achalasia: long-term outcome and predictors of response. Gastroenterology 110:1410–1415

Perkin GD, Murray-Lyon I (1998) Neurology and the gastrointestinal system. J Neurol Neurosurg Psychiatry 65:291–300

Ponce J, Garrigues V, Pertejo V et al. (1996) Individual prediction of response to pneumatic dilation in patients with achalasia. Dig Dis Sci 41:2135–2141

Pricolo VE, Park CS, Thompson WR (1993) Surgical repair of esophageal perforation due to pneumatic dilatation for achalasia. Is myotomy really necessary? Arch Surg 128:540–543 (discussion 543–544)

Saigal S, Kumar N (1996) Non-surgical treatment of achalasia cardia. Trop Gastroenterol 17:178–181

Schiano TD, Parkman HP, Miller LS et al. (1998) Use of botulinum toxin in the treatment of achalasia. Dig Dis 16:14–22

Schwartz HM, Cahow CE, Traube M (1993) Outcome after perforation sustained during pneumatic dilatation for achalasia. Dig Dis Sci 38:1409–1413

Shah SW, Khan AA, Alam A et al. (1998) Diffuse esophageal spasm: transforming into achalasia. JPMA J Pak Med Assoc 48:58–60

Shoenut JP, Duerksen D, Yaffe CS (1997) A prospective assessment of gastroesophageal reflux before and after treatment of achalasia patients: pneumatic dilation versus transthoracic limited myotomy. Am J Gastroenterol 92:1109–1112

Streitz JM Jr, Ellis FH Jr, Gibb SP et al. (1995) Achalasia and squamous cell carcinoma of the esophagus: analysis of 241 patients. Ann Thorac Surg 59:1604–1609

Sugarbaker DJ, Kearney DJ, Richards WG (1993) Esophageal physiology and pathophysiology. Surg Clin North Am 73:1101–1118

Topart P, Deschamps C, Taillefer R et al. (1992) Long-term effect of total fundoplication on the myotomized esophagus. Ann Thorac Surg 54:1046–1051 (discussion 1051–1052)

Vaezi MF, Richter JE (1998) Current therapies for achalasia: comparison and efficacy. J Clin Gastroenterol 27:21–35

Vaezi MF, Richter JE, Wilcox CM et al. (1999) Botulinum toxin versus pneumatic dilatation in the treatment of achalasia: a randomised trial. Gut 44:231–239

Walker SJ (1997) What's new in pathology, pathophysiology and management of benign esophageal disorders? Dis Esophagus 10:282–302

Wehrmann T, Jacobi V, Jung M et al. (1995) Pneumatic dilation in achalasia with a low-compliance balloon: results of a 5-year prospective evaluation. Gastrointest Endosc 42:31–36

Wehrmann T, Kokabpick H, Jacobi V, Seifert H, Lembcke B, Caspary WF (1999) Long-term results of endoscopic injection of botulinum toxin in elderly achalasic patients with tortuous megaesophagus or epiphrenic diverticulum. Endoscopy 31:352–358

Yoneyama F, Miyachi M, Nimura Y (1998) Manometric findings of the upper esophageal sphincter in esophageal achalasia. World J Surg 22:1043–1046

CHAPTER 4

Laparoscopic Cardiomyotomy for Achalasia

E. Hanisch, T. C. Schmandra, and A. Encke

Indications

Current indications for laparoscopic surgery include:
1. Primary therapy in the young
2. Failure of balloon dilation in individuals older than 40 years of age.

Contraindications

Contraindications for laparoscopic surgery include:
1. Severe chronic obstructive pulmonary disease
2. Previous upper abdominal surgery (relative)
3. Coagulopathy (e.g., in liver cirrhosis)
4. Malignant obstruction!
5. Gastroesophageal reflux with stricture formation
6. Diffuse esophageal spasms and nutcracker esophagus.

Techniques of Cardiomyotomy

The operating room set-up is similar to that for laparoscopic fundoplication. The surgeon stands between the legs of the patient with two assistants on the right and left side of the patient. An anti-Trendelenburg position is used (see Chap. 2, Figs. 2.1, 2.2).

The Veress needle is introduced at the umbilicus. The pneumoperitoneum is maintained at a maximal pressure of 12 mmHg.

The camera trocar is inserted halfway between the xiphoid process and the umbilicus. Three additional 12-mmHg trocars are placed: one located in the midline, just below the xiphoid process, one in the right hypochondrium below the costal margin, and one in the left lateral subcostal hypochondrium (Fig. 4.1).

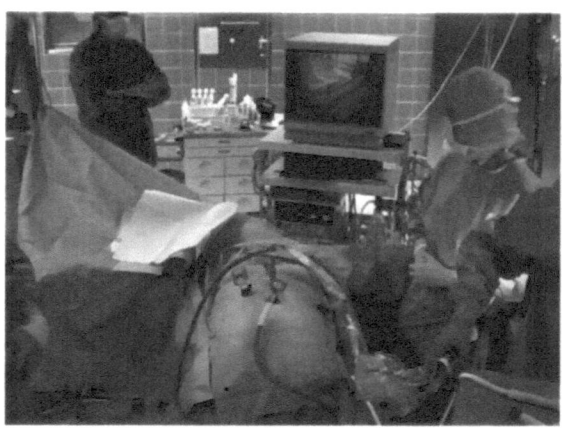

Fig. 4.1. Three additional 12-mmHg trocars are placed: one located in the midline, just below the xiphoid process, one in the right hypochondrium below the costal margin, and one in the left lateral subcostal hypochondrium

The left liver lobe is firstly lifted by a fan retractor (AutoSuture, Norwalk, Conn. USA) introduced via the subxiphoidal trocar.

The anterior distal esophagus is identified and longitudinal muscle fibers are bluntly separated and divided with the ultrasonic scalpel (Fig. 4.2a,b).

Transverse fibers are carefully separated from the underlying mucosa (Fig 4.3).

The myotomy is carried out proximally for about 5 cm from the gastroesophageal junction and distally onto the stomach for about 1–2 cm (Fig. 4.4).

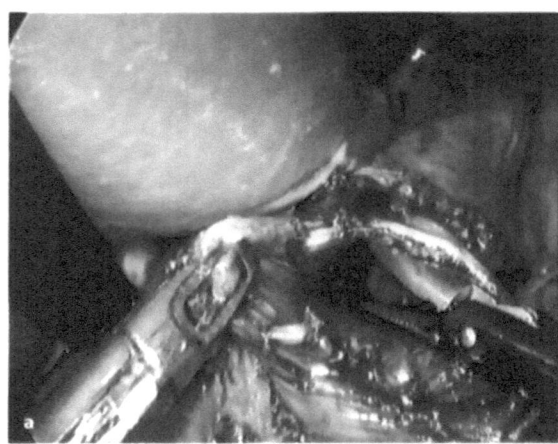

Fig. 4.2a,b. The anterior distal esophagus is identified and longitudinal muscle fibers are bluntly separated and divided

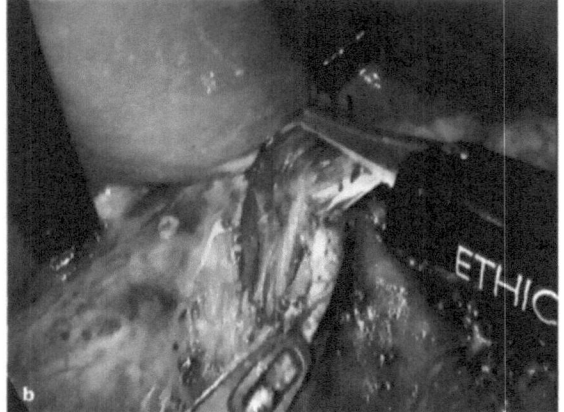

Fig. 4.2b

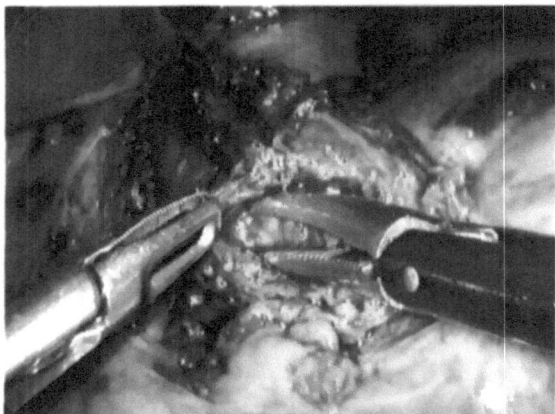

Fig. 4.3. Transverse fibers
are carefully separated
from the underlying
mucosa

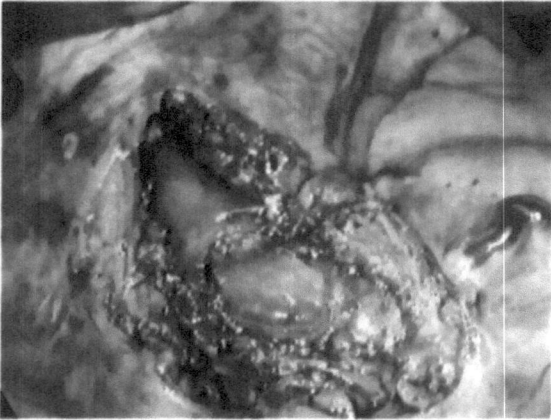

Fig. 4.4. The myotomy is
carried out proximally for
about 5 cm from the gas-
troesophageal junction
and distally onto the
stomach for about 1–2 cm

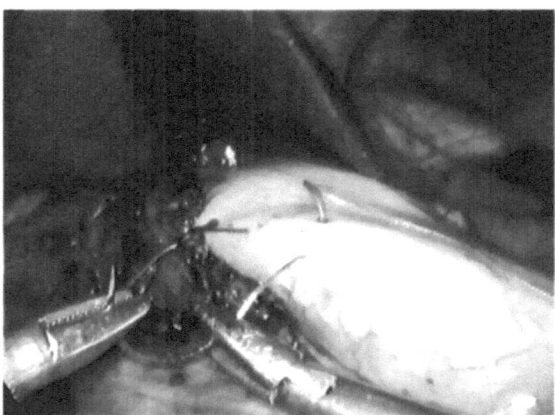

Fig. 4.5. The clearly bulging mucosa (muscle edges separated for approximately 40% of the esophageal circumference) is covered by an anterior hemifundoplication

Finally, the clearly bulging mucosa (muscle edges separated for approximately 40% of the esophageal circumference) is covered by an anterior hemifundoplication (Fig. 4.5).

To check for esophageal or gastric injuries at the end of the operation, the upper abdomen is covered with saline while the esophagus and stomach are carefully examined by a flexible endoscope.

Complications of Cardiomyotomy

1. Be aware that many failed myotomies stem from an incorrect preoperative diagnosis (rule out malignant secondary achalasia!).
2. Perforation of the mucosa is the most common complication and readily recognized, at least during air insufflation via the endoscope at the end of the operation. These injuries are easily repaired laparoscopically by single stitches.
3. Bleeding may occur from the liver (deploy fan retractor), anterior esophagus, or stomach when dissecting a fat pedicle.

Overall Results of Cardiomyotomy

Relief of dysphagia is achieved in 90%–100% of patients with an incidence of postoperative reflux of less than 10%.

References

Ellis F (1997) Failure after esophagomyotomy for esophageal motor disorders. Chest Surg Clin North Am 7:477–487

Emmermann A, Thonke F, Zornig C (1996) Die laparoskopische Kardiomyotomie bei Achalasie. Zentralbl Chir 121:303–306

Holzman M, Sharp K, Ladipo J, Eller R, Holcomb G, Richards W (1997) Laparoscopic surgical treatment of achalasia. Am J Surg 173:308–311

Hunter J, Trus Th, Branum G, Waring P (1997) Laparoscopic Heller myotomy and fundoplication for achalasia. Ann Surg 225:655–665

Oddsdottir M (1996) Laparoscopic management of achalasia. Surg Clin North Am 76:451–458

Raiser F, Hinder R, Swanstrom L, Filipi Ch, McBrideP, Katada N, Neary P (1996) Heller myotomy via minimal-access surgery. Arch Surg 131:593–598

Rosati R, Fumagalli U, Bona S (1998) Evaluating results of achalasia: recent advances in surgery. Surg Endosc 12:270–273

Spiess A, Kahrilas P (1998) Treating achalasia: from whalebone to laparoscope. JAMA 280:638–642

Trus T, Hunter J (1997) Minimal invasive surgery of the esophagus and stomach. Am J Surg 173:242–255

Vaezi M, Richter J (1998) Current therapies for achalasia: comparison and efficacy. J Clin Gastroenterol 27:21–35

Pathogenetic Aspects of Obesity

T. Konrad

Introduction

Obesity is considered to be the major nutritional disorder in many countries of the industrialized world. The physiology of the obese and their propensity for chronic disease has been of growing interest over the past few years. Overweight persons are at increased risk of coronary artery disease, arterial hypertension, and cancer. There is also a profound association between obesity, particularly intraabdominal adiposity, and the development of non-insulin-dependent diabetes mellitus (NIDDM). Obesity has reached epidemic proportions. This is paralleled by an increasing incidence of NIDDM. There is no doubt that weight gain and obesity are major clinical problems, which need to be prevented and managed more effectively.

Obesity is a heterogeneous disorder. When viewed in the broadest sense, it has been considered a disorder of energy balance. Nevertheless, the development of obesity in humans is of complex etiology, involving genetic and environmental components that affect regulatory and metabolic events. New concepts and techniques in endocrinology, neurobiology, genetics, and nutrition have yielded new insights into how environmental factors such as diet and physical expenditure interact to influence energy metabolism and body composition. The data from molecular genetics have clarified important sites of regulation of fat storage in humans. The pathogenesis of obesity has moved in recent decades from careful analysis of psychosocial factors to a deeper understanding of the biology of fat storage and energy metabolism. The psychological and behavioral aspects remain important because the final common act leading to either obesity or its amelioration is the individual's approach to altered food intake and/or physical activity.

The discovery of leptin, the product of the obese (*ob*) gene, has broadened the horizons of research into the regulation of body adiposity and energy balance. (Zhang et al. 1994). This hormone, produced exclusively

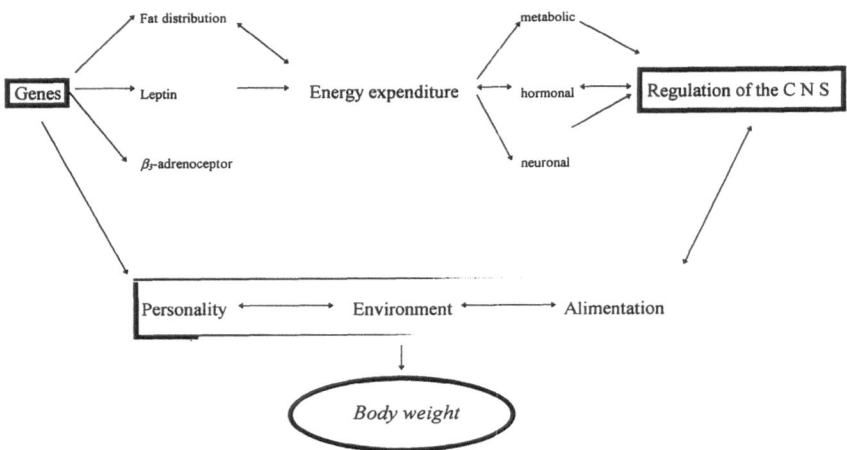

Fig. 5.1. Factors regulating body weight. *CNS*, central nervous system

by adipose tissue, conveys information to the brain on the size of energy stores and activates hypothalamic centers which regulate energy intake and expenditure. In addition, leptin affects several neuroendocrine mechanisms and regulates multiple hypothalamic – pituitary axes (Flier 1997). Thus, adipose tissue is not a simple fat storage depot, but also an important endocrine gland which produces a hormone that regulates body size. As early as in 1953, Kennedy first postulated this lipostatic theory of body weight control by the adipose tissue. Figure 5.1 summarizes the complex interplay between all these factors regulating body weight in humans.

Definition and Epidemiology

Visual inspection of a patient can give a subjective but fairly accurate estimate of the degree of obesity. Obesity is usually classified according to the body mass index (BMI, kg/m^2). Table 5.1 summarizes the different classes of body weight, ranging from low body weight to morbid adiposity. This simple measurement correlates quite strongly with other estimates of fatness, although some very muscular individuals may be classified as obese when they are not. The normal body weight is associated with the lowest risk of obesity-related diseases and the subsequent lowest mortality. The body weights of members of the general population can differ substantially. An individual's weight is generally relatively sta-

Table 5.1. Classification of body weight based on body mass index (BMI)

BMI (kg/m²)	
< 19	Low body weight
19 – 25	Normal body weight
25 – 30	Overweight
> 30	Obesity
> 40	Morbid obesity

Table 5.2. Incidence of overweight and obesity in industrialized countries

Country	Age (years)	Overweight (BMI 25 – 29) (%)		Adiposity (BMI > 30) (%)	
		Males	Females	Males	Females
Australia	25 – 64	44	25	12	13
Canada	18 – 74	41	23	15	15
Germany	25 – 74	51	45	17	19
Sweden	16 – 84	35	26	7	8
USA	> 20	39	25	18	23

ble. Individual body weight variance is typically only 0.5% over periods of 6 – 10 weeks (Keesey and Hirvonen 1997). Andres and coworkers (1985) found that body weight increases with age and they recommend maintaining a lower BMI for younger persons (19 – 25 kg/m²) and for persons above 50 years a BMI between 23 – 29 kg/m². It should be mentioned, however, that cardiovascular morbidity and mortaliy increases above a BMI of 25 kg/m², as clearly shown by the Framingham study (Hubert et al. 1983) and the Nurses' Health Study (Manson et al. 1995).

The clinical diagnosis of obesity is easy to verify, but other diseases related with obesity must nevertheless be excluded, i.e., hypothyreoidism, Cushing disease, polycystic ovarian syndrome, and other affections of the hypothalamus and hypophysis. A number of rare genetic diseases are associated with obesity, but through unknown mechanisms: the Prader-Willi syndrome, the Laurence-Moon-Biedl syndrome, Alstrom's syndrome, the Cohen syndrome, the Carpenter syndrome, and Blount's disease (see textbooks on genetic disorders for further description). Drugs, such as antidepressive and neuroleptic drugs, can also promote increases in body weight (see Table 5.1).

It is thought that a significant contributing factor to obesity in modern industrialized societies is the abundant and varied supply of palatable, high-fat foods. Although regional and cultural factors may still have a predominant impact on nutrition and increase in body weight, the worldwide fast-food wave may smooth ethnological differences, finally creating a global standard malnutrition with fat. Table 5.2 summarizes the incidence of overweight and obesity in five industrialized countries. In Germany, every second person is overweight and every fifth suffers from morbid adiposity (Hoffmeister et al. 1994).

Genetic Aspects

Central or visceral obesity is common and associated with hypertension, dyslipidemia, insulin resistance, diabetes, and premature death from cardiovascular disease and cancers such as breast and endometrium. The accumulation of intraabdominal fat rather than subcutaneous fat is associated more with these disease processes (Bjorntorp 1991; Kohort et al. 1993). Epidemiological studies (Bouchard et al. 1991, 1996) point to a genetic contribution of abdominal and subcutaneous fat distribution. These data have yielded heritability estimates of 25% – 45% of the individual differences in BMI or body fat. Moreover, Carey et al. (1996) demonstrated in twins that the variance of central fat distribution is approximately 70% genetically determined.

Glucocorticoids are thought to play a pivotal role in the pathogenesis of central obesity. This is convincing since Cushing's syndome is clinically characterized by an increase in the size of intraabdominal fat stores compared with subcutaneous fat (Rebuffe-Scrive et al. 1988). Adipose stroma cells from omental fat, but not subcutaneous fat, can generate active cortisol from inactive cortisone through the expression of 11β-hydroxysteroid dehydrogenase enzyme (Bujalska et al. 1997). In vivo, such a mechanism would cause a constant exposure of glucocorticoid specifically to omental adipose tissue. Therefore, as suggested by Bujalska et al. (1997), central obesity may reflect "Cushing's disease of the omentum". The genetic expression and distribution of *glucocorticoid receptor* in visceral adipose tissue also determines the extent of the central fat accumulation (Ottoson et al. 1994).

β_3-Adrenoceptor gene mutation is also associated with abdominal obesity and insulin resistance and an increased capacity to weight gain (Clement et al. 1995). Hoffstedt et al. (1996) demonstrated for the first time a relationship between upper-body obesity and visceral adipocyte β_3-adrenoceptor sensitivity. A higher sensitivity of adrenoceptor of the fat tissue may therefore result in a higher susceptibility to catecholamines, which may then enhance lipolysis with a higher delivery of nonesterified free fatty acids (NEFA) into the portal circulation. Thus, higher β_3-adrenoceptor activity may represent a link between central adiposity and adverse effects of NEFA on liver function, including impaired metabolism of glucose, lipoproteins, and insulin. In contrast to these findings in obese non-diabetic men, a mutation of β_3-adrenoceptor appears to be responsible for the onset of NIDDM (Walston et al. 1995): a lower expression of this gene would be followed by a lower lipolysis and reduced thermogenesis, finally leading to an increase in body weight and a decrease of insulin sensitivity.

Leptin is the peptide produce of the *ob* gene. The genetically obese *ob/ob* mouse produces a defective leptin, resulting in massive obesity and hyperphagia. In addition to obesity, the *ob/ob* mouse has insulin-resistant diabetes and defects in fat metabolism, thermogenesis, and reproduction (Zhang et al. 1994). The human homologue protein is also exclusively secreted from adipose tissue and is 84% homologous to the mouse protein. Therefore, the question arises whether obesity in humans could be caused by leptin deficiency. Clinical studies, howewer, failed to describe any mutations of the leptin gene (Considine et al. 1995; Maffei et al. 1996; Niki et al. 1996). The secretion of leptin from adipose tissue in the circulation is pulsatile and follows a circardian rhythm, with highest levels observed at night (Licinio et al. 1997). Serum leptin concentrations in humans exhibit a sexual dimorphism, with higher levels in women than in men (Havel et al. 1996). The reproductive hormone status may account in part for this dimorphism. This suggestion was supported by the finding that a negative association exists between serum testosterone and serum leptin levels (Jockenhovel et al. 1997).

Both body adiposity and acute changes in energy balance appear to regulate leptin expression and levels; however, the precise mechanism remains to be elucidated: Leptin expression and levels increase as the size of the adipose tissue triglyceride stores increase (Maffei et al. 1996; Niki et al. 1996). An increase in caloric intake results in a sharp increase in serum leptin, approximately 40% over baseline within 12 h, in the absence of changes in body weight. In contrast, serum leptin concentrations in humans do not increase acutely in the postprandial state (Kolacynski et al. 1996a). On the other hand, both leptin expression and levels decline rapidly in response to starvation (Kolacynski et al. 1996b). In vitro and in vivo studies point to positive effects of insulin (Rentsch and Chiesi 1996), glucocorticoids (Wabitsch et al. 1996), and cytokines (Mantzoros et al. 1997) on leptin expression and secretion. There is no effect of leptin on glucose transport and insulin action in adipose and muscle cells (Ranganathan et al. 1998). Leptin, however, indirectly suppresses glucose-induced insulin secretion and stimulates hypoglycemia-induced glucagon secretion through activation of the sympathetic nervous system (Mizuno et al. 1998).

Intracerebroventricular administration of leptin results in a more potent response, i.e., weight loss, compared with the response to systemic administration, suggesting that the central nervous system (CNS) is the major site of action of leptin (Schwartz et al. 1996). The existence of a saturable transport system for leptin across the blood – brain barrier, presumably in the choroid plexus and the hypothalamus (Banks et al. 1996), support this suggestion. Leptin has been shown to decrease the release of the biological "appetizer" neuropeptide Y (NPY) in vitro and hypothalamic levels in vivo (Stephens et al. 1995; Wang et al. 1997). High NPY concentrations in this area inhibit sympathetic nervous system outflow, and decrease energy expenditure and improved storage of fat (Schwartz and Seeley 1997). Prolonged NPY receptor blockade with a newly developed antagonist (Criscione et al. 1998) causes an initial fall in food intake in free-feeding rats which then becomes progressively attenuated over time. Although food intake returns to normal with prolonged NPY receptor blockade, body weight remains low. These findings suggest that NPY antagonists have a role to play in the treatment of obesity.

Leptin levels increase accordingly in response to body adiposity in both adults and children (Considine et al. 1996; Hassink et al. 1996). This

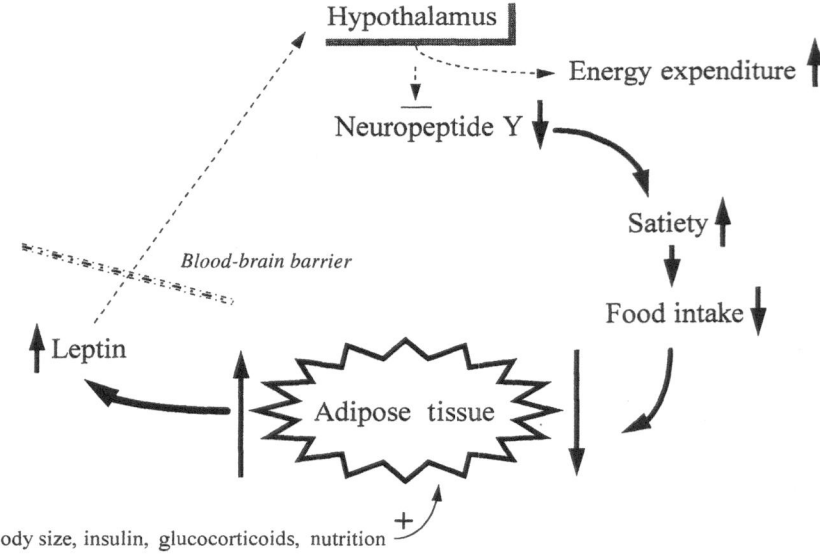

Fig. 5.2. Overview of leptin, its regulation, and effects

observation has suggested that most cases of human obesity are associated with leptin resistance (Considine et al. 1996). A decreased cerebrospinal fluid/serum leptin ratio suggests that a readily saturable putative transport mechanism across the blood – brain barrier may account for the apparent leptin resistance in obese patients (Caro et al. 1996). A modest hypoadrenocorticism in association with obesity may also be responsible for the leptin resistance in obese subjects (Caro et al. 1996).

Starvation (Fig. 5.2) is another condition where leptin plays an important role. Under such conditions, a sharp decline in leptin levels occurs which is disproportionate to body adiposity changes (Wang et al. 1997). Thus, an acute drop in serum leptin levels could be responsible for the documented decrease in energy expenditure that accompanies weight loss (Leibel et al. 1995). Such changes in energy expenditure may account for the clinically observed difficulty that obese people face when attempting to lose weight. This finding creates the impression that the body may be employing leptin as a rapidly acting defence mechanism that aims to maintain the "status quo" of energy balance and body size.

Energy Expenditure: A Hypothalamic Function

The coordinated control of energy intake and expenditure is the only way to maintain a stable level of body weight. It is often the case, however, that control of intake is insufficient to account for the stability of body weight. In these cases, a reduced rate of energy expenditure appears to be responsible for the body weight gain. Ravussin et al. (1988) could clearly show that these differences in energy expenditure and thermogenesis are hereditary. This observation may explain why increases in food intake frequently fail to produce the changes in body weight expected on the basis of the caloric excess or deficit. The weight losses produced by most diets are typically less than those expected from the apparent caloric deficit.

Experimental studies of genetically-transmitted and diet-induced forms of obesity in animals similarly suggest a view of obesity as a condition of body energy regulation at an elevated "set-point" (Keesey and Hirvonen 1997). The concept of a set point of body weight suggests that each person has a control system that "sets" how much weight, or alternatively how much fat, he or she should have. An individual's set point is apparently adjustable, shifting over a lifespan in conjunction with naturally occurring, but still unspecific, physiologic changes. It appears that hypothalamic mechanisms play a primary role in setting the level at which individuals regulate body weight. Serotonin and noradrenaline act synergistically in the regulation of energy expenditure. A novel anti-obesity drug, the serotonin and noradrenaline re-uptake inhibitor sibutramine, increases energy expenditure in rats (Heal et al. 1998). This sibutramine-induced thermogenesis is mediated by a selective sympathetic activation of brown adipose tissue, and it is also a centrally mediated effect because it can be abolished by pretreating the animals with a specific ganglionic blocker.

Approaches to Weight Control: Diet, Exercise, Drugs

The "set-point" theory suggests that people are at a given weight because they are "set" there. That is, one's set point is the weight one normally maintains. Set-point theory has been used to suggest that weight loss programs are misguided and that the effort to lose weight is inevitably fraught with failure because a set point will bring individuals back up to their pre-weightloss weight. Therefore, it is to be expected that an individual with a regulated form of obesity will display natural resistance to diet-induced weight loss. Compensatory metabolic adjustments to caloric restriction will not only diminish initial weight loss, but facilitate the restoration of weight previously lost. Sustained weight reduction, if achieved by dieting, will therefore require a lifelong commitment to a daily caloric intake not only less than satisfying, but possibly lower than that of individuals of normal body weight (Table 5.3).

These partly theoretical considerations of weight reduction in overweight subjects may explain the difficulty associated with definitively treating obesity. In other words: Therapy of obesity is a lifelong treatment of a chronic disease. Therefore, crash diets for a few days or weeks generally accomplish few permanent results. Because of the long-term requirement for a diet, any diet must be tailored to the individual's tastes

Dietary regimen[a]	**Table 5.3.** Different approaches to the therapy of obesity . [Modified from Hauner (1997)]
– Fat-reduced diet	
– Caloric-reduced diet	
– Very low caloric diet	
– Vegetarian diet	

[a] Dietary regimens may also include one or more of the following: modification of behavior, excercise programs, anti-obesity drugs, and surgical treatment.

and habits. The overall guideline for nutrition therapy is that the diet must be adequate: It is not possible to calculate a diet under 1100 calories that contains adequate amounts of vitamins and minerals. The goal of weight loss is to lose as much fat as possible while losing as little lean mass as possible. A mixed, balanced diet is a sensible approach to long-term weight reduction (Hauner 1997). Very low calorie diets severely limit daily intake to 300–700 calories. Some diets are stricly limited to protein and have been called protein-supplemented modified fasts (PMSF). The extra weight lost early in the diet when protein alone is given is that of water. With this water diuresis, there is also electrolyte loss as well. Therefore, adequate supplementation with vitamins and minerals is mandatory. Moreover, it is dangerous to perform this type of diet over a period of more than 12 weeks, since side effects such as orthostatic hypotension secondary to both sodium loss and impaired norepinephrine secretion, fatigue, and cold intolerance due to rapid fat loss may occur. The heavier the patient, the safer the diet must be. The lighter the patient, the more lean body mass is lost per unit weight loss, so that more caution, more liberal calories, and a shorter time period of diet should be followed (Hauner 1997). In every case, weight loss of about 5%–10% of body weight over 6–12 months should be the aim of every dietary therapy, which must be followed by maintenance for 1 year of the reduced body weight achieved. In those patients in which obesity (BMI >30 kg/m^2) has caused severe physical complications, a very low diet is required. Behavior modification and increasing physical activity must accompany this therapy. Administration of anti-obesity drugs may also be helpful in such patients.

The most difficult problem after successful weight reduction is the maintenance of a reduced body weight. The ability to maintain weight loss may depend on the severity of obesity and the amount of hypercellularity of the adipocytes in a given individual. Therefore, in those patients with morbid obesity (BMI >30 kg/m^2), a maintenance of the reduced body weight is difficult to achieve.

Conclusions

Although a huge number of experimental and clinical studies have broadened our knowledge about leptin in the regulation of body weight, the precise physiological mechanisms of this adipose hormone are not clearly understood. After the enthusiasm that followed the discovery of leptin and the hope of definitively treating obesity, disillusionment has now set in among most of the research groups. Furthermore, the therapeutic potential of leptin as observed in *ob/ob* mice has still to be established in humans. New anti-obesity drugs, however, are on the way, which may interfere with the complex hypothalamic regulation of satiety, energy expenditure, and other important hypothalamic – pituitary activities.

References

Andres R, Elahi D, Tobin JDet al. (1985) Impact of age on weight goals. Ann Intern Med 103:1030 – 1033

Banks WA, Kastin AJ, Huang W et al. (1996) Leptin enters the brain by a saturable system independent of insulin. Peptides 17:305 – 311

Bjorntorp P (1991) Metabolic implications of body fat distribution. Diabetes Care 14:1132 – 1143

Bouchard C, Despres JP, Mauriege P et al. (1991) The genes in the constellation of determinants of regional fat distribution. Int J Obesity 15:8 – 18

Bouchard C, Rice T, Lemieux S et al. (1996) Major gene for abdominal visceral fat area in the Quebec Family Study. Int J Obesity 20:420 – 427

Bujalska IJ, Kumar S, Stewart PM (1997) Does central obesity reflect "Cushing's disease of the omentum"? Lancet 349:1210 – 1213

Carey DGP, Nguyen TV, Campbell LV et al. (1996) Genetic influences on central abdominal fat: a twin study. Int J Obesity 20:722 – 726

Caro JF, Kolacynski JW, Nyce MR et al. (1996) Decreased cerebrospinal fluid/serum leptin ratio in obesity: a possible mechanism for leptin resistance. Lancet 348:159 – 161

Clement K, Vaisse C, Manning BS et al. (1995) Genetic variation in the β_3-adrenergic receptor and increased capacity to gain weight in patients with morbid obesity. New Engl J Med 333:352 – 354

Considine RV, Considine EL, Williams CJ et al. (1995) Evidence against either a premature stop codon or the absence of obese gene mRNA in human obesity. J Clin Invest 95:2986 – 2988

Considine RV, Sinha MK, Heiman ML et al. (1996) Serum immunoreactive-leptin concentrations in normal-weight and obese humans. N Engl J Med 334:292 – 295

Criscione L, Rigollier C, Batzl-Hartmann C et al. (1998) Food intake in free-feeding and energy-deprived lean rats is mediated by the neuropetide Y_5 receptor. J Clin Invest 102:2136 – 2145

Flier JS (1997) Leptin expression and action: new experimental paradigms. Proc Nat Acad Sci 94:4242 – 4245

Hassink SG, Sheslow DV, de Lancey E et al. (1996) Serum leptin in children with obesity: in relation to gender and development. Pediatrics 98:201 – 203

Hauner H (1997) Strategien der Adipositastherapie. Internist 3:244 – 250

Havel PJ, Kasim-Karakas S, Dubuc GR et al. (1996) Gender differences in leptin concentrations. Nat Med 2:949 – 950

Heal DJ, Aspley S, Prow MR et al. (1998) Sibutramine: a novel anti-obesity drug. A review of the pharmacological evidence to differentiate it from d-amphetamine and Dd-fenfluramine. Int J Obes 22:18S-28S

Hoffmeister M, Mensink GBM, Stolzenberg H (1994) National trends and risk factors for cardiovascular disease in Germany. Prev Med 23:197–205

Hoffstedt J, Wahrenberg H, Thörne A et al. (1996) The metabolic syndrome is related to β_3-adrenoceptor sensitvity in visceral adipose tissue. Diabetologia 39:838–844

Hubert HB, Feinlieb M, McNamara PM et al. (1983) Obesity as an independent risk factor for cardiovascular disease: a 26-year follow-up of participants in the Framingham heart study. Circulation 67:968–977

Jockenhovel F, Blum WF, Vogel E et al. (1997) Testosterone substitution normalizes elevated serum leptin levels in the hypogonadal men. J Clin Endocrinol Metab 82:2510–2513

Keesey RE, Hirvonen MD (1997) Body weight set-points: determination and adjustment. J Nutr 127:1875S-1883S

Kennedy GR (1953) The role of depot tat in the hypothalamic control of food intake in the rat. Proc R Soc 140:578–597

Kohort WM, Kirwan JP, Staten MA et al. (1993) Insulin resistance in aging is related to abdominal obesity. Diabetes 42:273–281

Kolacynski JW, Ohannesian J, Considine RV et al. (1996) Response of leptin to short-term and prolonged over feeding in humans. J Clin Endocrinol Metab 81:4162–4165

Kolacynski JW, Considine RV, Ohannesian J et al. (1996) Response of leptin to short-term fasting and refeeding in humans: a link with ketogenesis but not with ketones themselves. Diabetes 45:1511–1515

Leibel RL, Rosenbaun M, Hirsch J (1995) Changes in energy expenditure resulting from altered body weight. N Engl J Med 332:621–628

Licinio J, Mantzoros C, Negrao AB et al. (1997) Human leptin levels are pulsatile and inversely related to pituitary-adrenal function. Nat Med 3:575–579

Maffei M, Halaas J, Ravussin E et al. (1995) Leptin levels in human and rodent: measurement of plasma leptin and ob mRNA in obese and weight reduced subjects. Nat Med 1:1155–1161

Maffei M, Stoffel M, Barone M et al. (1996) Absence of mutations in the human OB gene in obese/diabetic individuals. Diabetes 45:679–682

Manson JE, Willett WC, Stampfer MJ et al. (1995) Body weight and mortality among women. N Engl J Med 333:677–685

Mantzoros CS, Moschos S, Avramopoulos I et.al. (1997) Leptin concentrations in relation to BMI and activation of the TNF alpha systems. J Clin Endocrinol Metab 82:3408–3413

Mizuno A, Murakami T, Otani S et al. (1998) Leptin affects pancreatic endocrine functions through the sympathetic nervous system. Endocrinology 139:3863–3870

Niki T, Mori H, Tamori Y et al. (1996) Human obese gene: molecular screening in Japanese and Asian Indian NIDDM patients associated with obesity. Diabetes 45:675–678

Ottoson M, Vikman-Adolfsson K, Enerbäck S et al. (1994) The effect of cortisol on the regulation of lipoprotein lipase activity in human adipose tissue. J Clin Endocrinol Metab 79:820–825

Ranganathan S, Ciaraldi TP, Henry RR et al. (1998) Lack of effect of leptin on glucose transport, lipoprotein lipase, and insulin action in adipose and muscle cells. Endocrinology 139:2509–2513

Ravussin E, Lillioja S, Knowler WC et al. (1998) Reduced rate of energy expenditure as a risk factor for body weight gain. N Engl J Med 318:467–472

Rebuffe-Scrive M, Krotkiewski M, Elfersson J et al. (1988) Muscle and adipose tissue morphology in Cushing's syndrome. J Clin Endocrinol Metab 67:1122–1125

Rentsch J, Chiesi M (1996) Regulation of ob gene mRNA levels in cultured adipocytes. FEBS Lett 379:55–59

Schwartz MW, Seeley RJ (1997) Neuroendocrine response to starvation and weight loss. N Engl J Med 336:1802–1811

Schwartz MW, Seeley RJ, Campfield LA et al. (1996) Identification of targets of leptin action in rat hypothalamus. J Clin Invest 98:1101–1106

Stephens TW, Basinski M, Bristow PK et al. (1995) The role of neuropeptide Y in the antiobesity action of the obese gene product. Nature 377:530–532

Wabitsch M, Jensen PB, Blum WF et al. (1996) Insulin and cortisol promote leptin production in cultured human fat cells. Diabetes 45:1435–1438

Walston J, Silver K, Bogardus C et al. (1995) Time of onset of non-insulin-dependent diabetes mellitus and genetic variation in the β_3-adrenergic receptor gene. N Engl J Med 333:343–347

Wang Q, Bing C, Al-Barazanji K et al. (1997) Interactions between leptin and the hypothalamic neuropeptide Y neurons in the control of food intake and energy homeostasis. Diabetes 46:335–361

Zhang Y, Proenca R, Maffei M et al. (1994) Positional cloning of the mouse obese gene and its human homologue. Nature 372:425–432

Adjustable Silicone Gastric Banding

E. Hanisch, T. C. Schmandra, and A. Encke

Indications

1. Patients having failed to achieve weight reduction with non-surgical measures (dietary regimens, psychological assistance, motion-based therapy) and who are motivated to ensure a positive and lasting post-surgery result (active participation in treatment and long-term follow up).
2. A body mass index (BMI) greater than 40 kg/m^2 indicates the patient as a potential candidate for surgical treatment.
3. Patients with a BMI of between 35 and 40 kg/m^2 may be considered for surgical therapy if they show high-risk co-morbid conditions (e.g., cardiopulmonary problems, severe diabetes mellitus, joint disease).

Contraindications

1. Carefully rule out that patients are sweet-eaters.
2. Patients with severe psychological or psychiatric disorders are poor candidates.
3. Patients older than 50 years should be considered at higher risk of complications.
4. Neuroendocrine causes of obesity need to be ruled out (e.g., Cushing's syndrome).

Surgical Technique

1. *Positioning of the patient:* To enable a laparoscopic procedure of gastric banding, the patient is placed in a moderate 30° reversed Trendelenburg tilt to displace the intraabdominal organs downwards, thus improving access to the proximal stomach. The patient's thighs are fully abducted and slightly flexed. The surgeon stands between the patient's legs, the first assistant on the patient's right side and the second assistant on the left (Fig. 6.1).

2. *Pneumoperitoneum:* Pneumoperitoneum is achieved through a Verress needle which is introduced in the left upper quadrant. In case of former abdominal surgery, introduction is performed via minimal laparotomy in a midline supraumbilical position. Carbon dioxide is used as the insufflation gas. Intraabdominal pressure is maintained at 16 mmHg.

3. *Placement of trocars:* The laparoscopic procedure is performed via four trocars (12 mm). The first trocar is placed in a median supraumbilical position. The best site should be the mid-point of the xyphoumbilical line. After insertion of a 30° optical system, inspection of the intraabdominal organs should be performed. The other trocars are then placed under visual control: one just below the xiphoid process to insert the liver retractor, and two in a subcostal position of the right and left upper quadrant of the abdomen for laparoscopic instruments (Fig. 6.2).

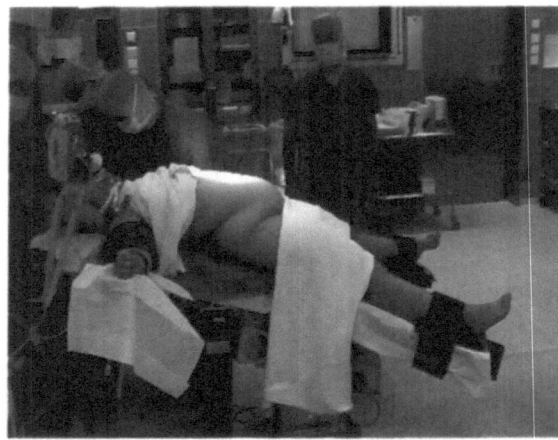

Fig. 6.1. Positioning of the patient

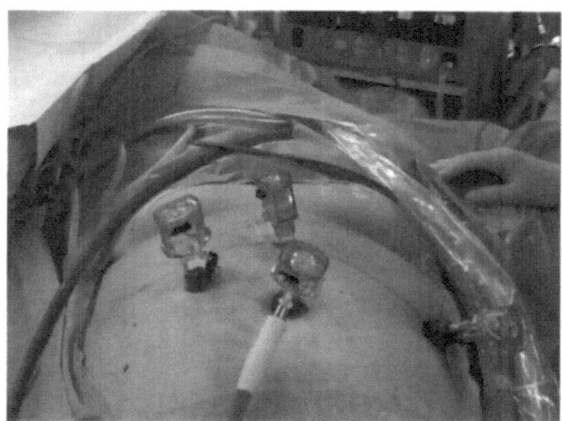

Fig. 6.2. Placement of trocars

4. *Exposure of the region of interest:* After introduction of the liver retractor, the gastric region is thoroughly exposed. The anesthesiologist then inserts a special calibration tube into the patient's stomach. The tube is characterized by an inflatable balloon catheter with a pressure sensor at its tip. The anesthesiologist fills the balloon with 20 ml room air. Under visual control, the tube is pulled back from the antrum to the gastroesophageal junction, determining the future gastric pouch size, the position of the gastric band, and the levels where dissection of the lesser and greater curvature needs to be performed.

5. *Dissection of the lesser curvature:* After deflation of the balloon and withdrawal of the calibration tube into the esophagus, the lesser curvature is dissected at the determined level (i.e. distal to the 20 ml ballon; description see above) with the Ultracision (Ethicon Endo-Surgery, Cincinatti, Ohio, USA) instrument. Opening and further dissection of the hepatogastric ligament should be narrow and performed as close as possible to the stomach wall in order to minimize the risk of band (and/or stomach) slippage. Visual control is obligatory for the entire dissection of the hepatogastric ligament. The posterior stomach wall should be clearly visible. For safer blunt dissection, we additionally use a special "snap-off" splaying instrument (Hourlay Autostatic Retractor, Duchateau, Rouvreux, Belgium). During laparoscopic preparation, care should be taken not to damage the gastric wall, retrogastric vessels, or the nerve of Latarjet (Figs. 6.3a – d).

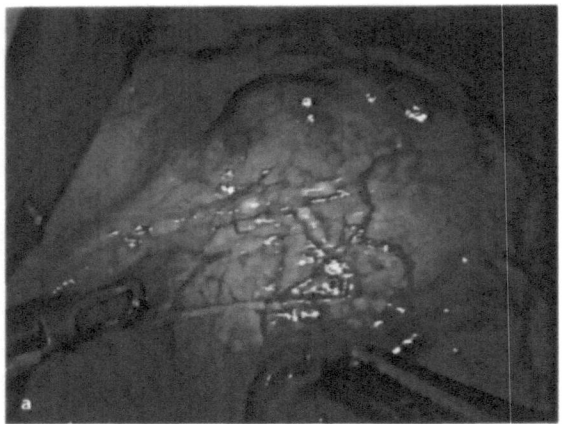

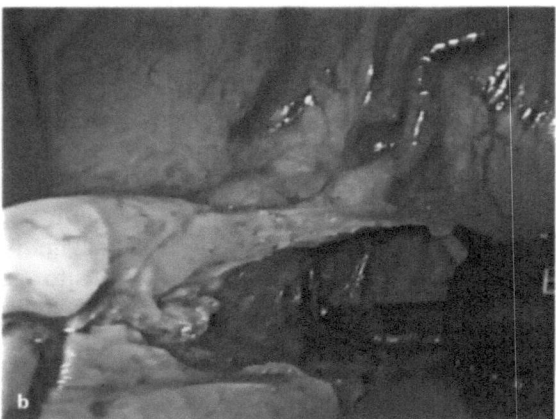

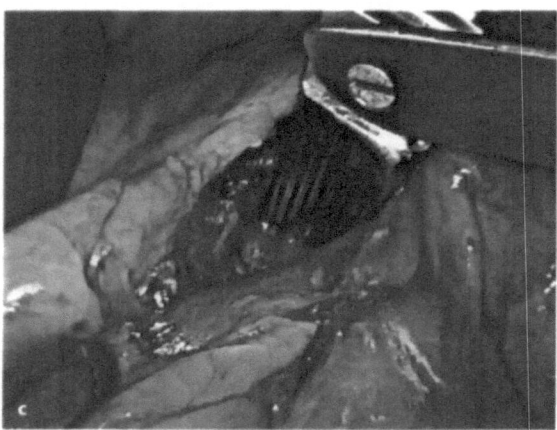

Fig. 6.3a – e. Dissection of
the lesser curvature

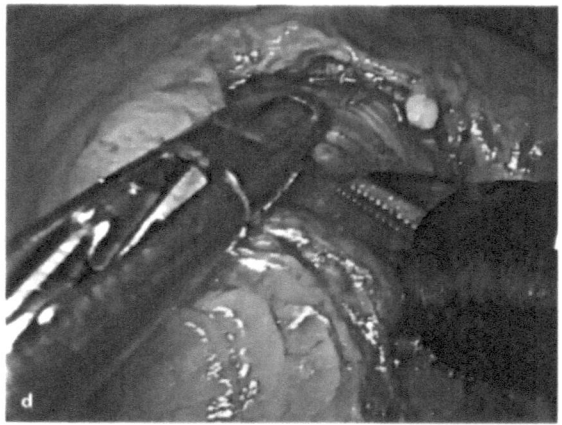

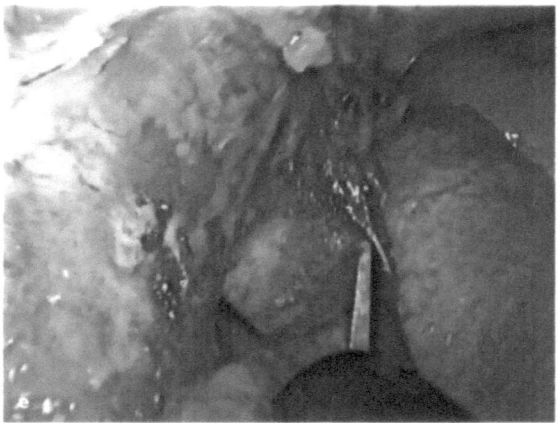

Fig. 6.3d, e

6. *Dissection of the greater curvature:* Dissection of the gastrophrenic ligament starts just proximal to the short gastric vessels, which should not be damaged (Fig. 6.3e). Dissection is performed with the gastrophrenic ligament under tension, pulling the stomach fundus caudally. Again, dissection into the gastrophrenic ligament should be narrow and close to the gastric wall to avoid silicone-band slippage.

7. *Retrogastric tunnelization:* A special grasping and rotating instrument (Roticulator Endograsp, AutoSuture, Norwalk, Conn., USA) is needed for the retrogastric passage joining both dissected areas. The

Roticulator is first introduced into the dissection of the lesser curvature and then gently pushed towards the gastrophrenic opening. As far as possible, tunnelization should be performed under visual control. By gently curving and rotating the instrument, its tip becomes visible as it points out through the opening of the greater curvature. The Roticulator should be left in the tunnel while introducing the silicone band. To avoid intraabdominal damage, the tip of the rotating instrument should grasp the peritoneal sheath of the diaphragm (Fig. 6.4). Before insertion and placement of the silicone band, the upper abdominal cavity is filled with saline solution. Air is insufflated into the stomach via a nasal tube to detect any possible perforation of the posterior gastric wall.

8. *Insertion and placement of the silicone band:* The anesthesiologist again introduces the calibrating tube into the patient's stomach. The balloon catheter (representing the gastric pouch size) is filled with 20 ml saline solution and withdrawn to the gastroesophageal junction. The calibration tube is now connected with an electronic sensor system (Gastrostenometer, BioEnterics, Carpinteria, Calif., USA). The pressure level sensed by the tip of the tube is represented in the number of sequential lights activated on the Gastrostenometer's display. We now temporarily remove the trocar in the left upper quadrant which is too small for band introduction. The trocar site is immediately probed (under video control) with the surgeon's finger (Fig. 6.5a) to prevent air loss. Via this canal, the checked and prepared silicone band (BioEnterics, Carpinteria, Calif.) is introduced intra-

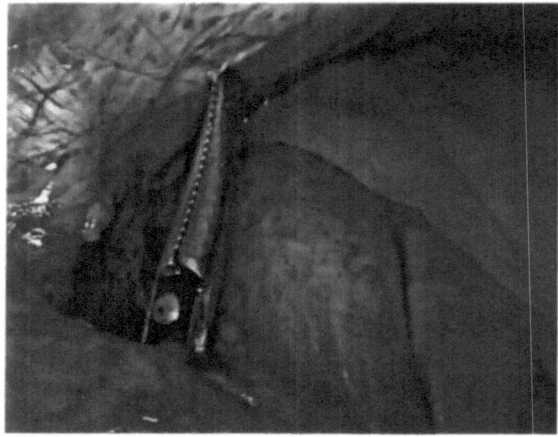

Fig. 6.4. Retrogastric tunnelization

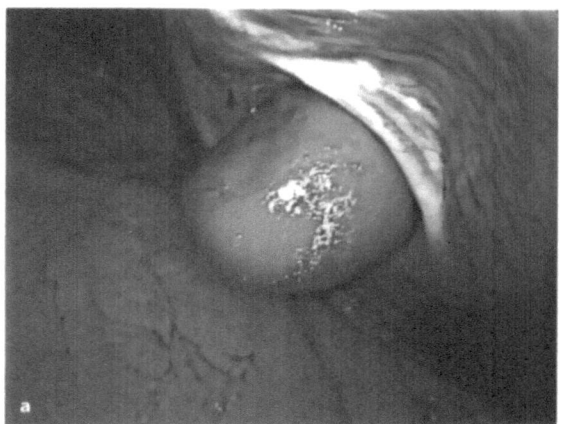

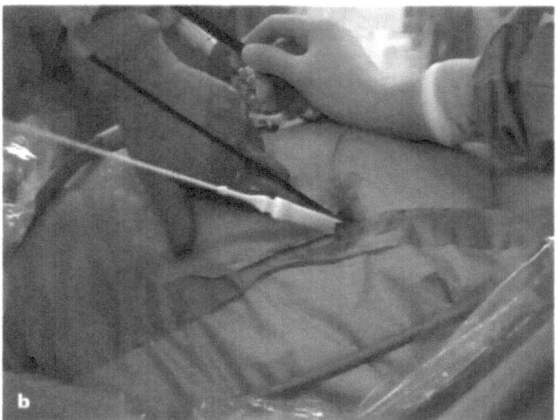

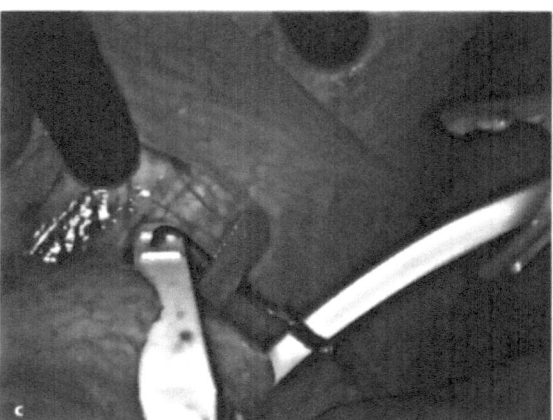

Fig. 6.5a – c. Insertion and placement of the silicone band

peritoneally (Fig. 6.5b). Following introduction of the band, the removed trocar is re-inserted in its former site in the left upper quadrant. Intraperitoneally, the band's end plug is grasped by the Roticulator, drawn through the retrogastric tunnel, and placed around the stomach at the level of dissection (Fig. 6.5c). The position is checked in regard to the calibration balloon.

9. *Closure and tightening of the silicone band:* The tubing of the silicone band is introduced into the buckle and the system is tightened. The closure instrument is then inserted via the trocar into the left upper quadrant. By correct use of the instrument, an adequate locking of the band is achieved (Figs. 6.6a,b). On the Gastrostenometer's display,

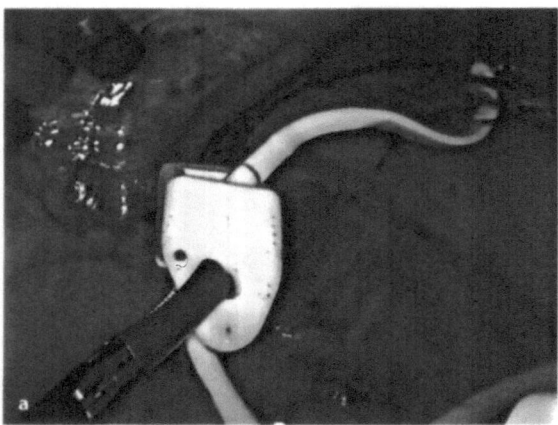

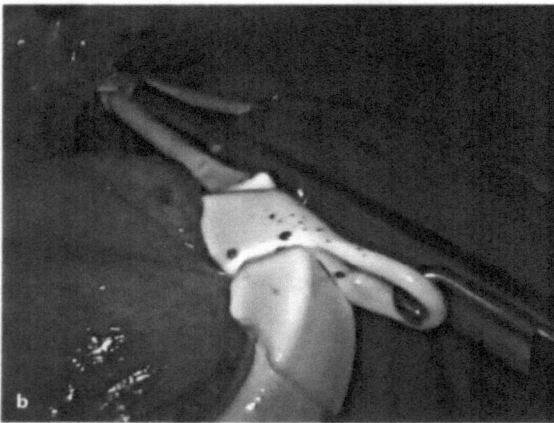

Fig. 6.6a,b. Closure and tightening of the silicone band

one or two lights are illuminated to confirm correct band-locking. The end of the tubing is then grasped with laparoscopic forceps and drawn outside the abdomen through the trocar in the left upper quadrant.

10. *Calibration of the adjustable silicone gastric band:* To calibrate the gastric pouch stoma, sterile saline solution is now injected into an inflatable portion of the adjustable silicone band. This is performed with a syringe connected to the end of the tubing which lies outside the abdomen. With increasing filling of the inflatable portion, the stoma diameter of the gastric pouch becomes smaller. This can be measured by the pressure sensor in the tip of the calibration tube in the stomach. On the Gastrostenometer, the sequential lights are displaced to the right. Illumination of the fourth light on the display corresponds to the intended pouch stoma of 12 mm. This is achievable with a filling volume of 2–4 ml saline solution. Outside the abdomen, the band's tubing is temporarily double-clamped with rubber-shod clamps. The calibration tube inside the stomach is removed after total deflation.

11. *Stabilization of the gastric band with retention sutures:* To prevent the silicone band from slipping, two seromuscular stitches are placed just proximal to and distal of the band. Suturing directly above the band's buckle should be avoided to minimize the risk of stomach perforation. The surgeon should be careful not to suture the silicone band to the stomach (Figs. 6.7a,b).

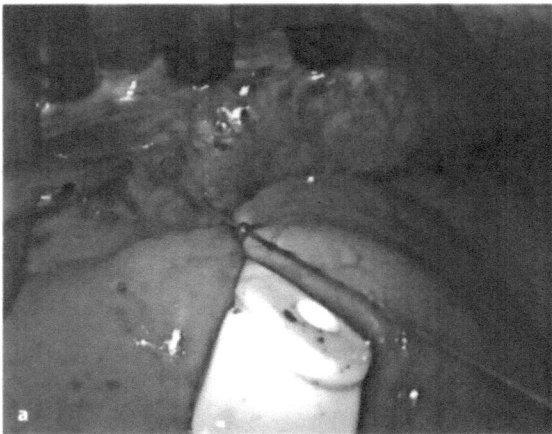

Fig. 6.7a,b. Stabilization of the gastric band with retention sutures

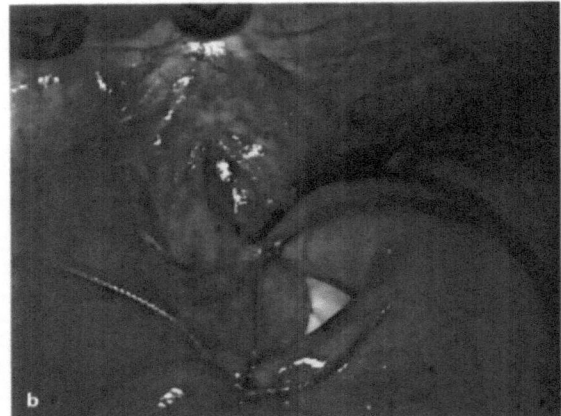

Fig. 6.7b

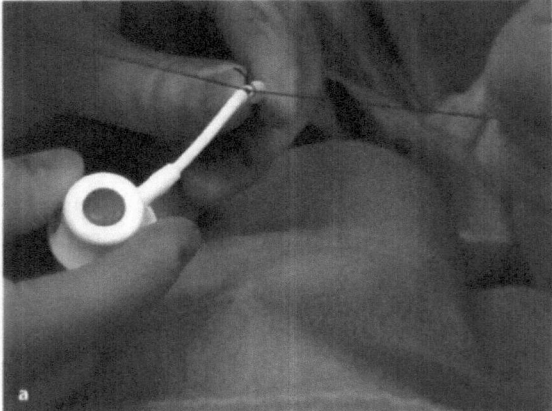

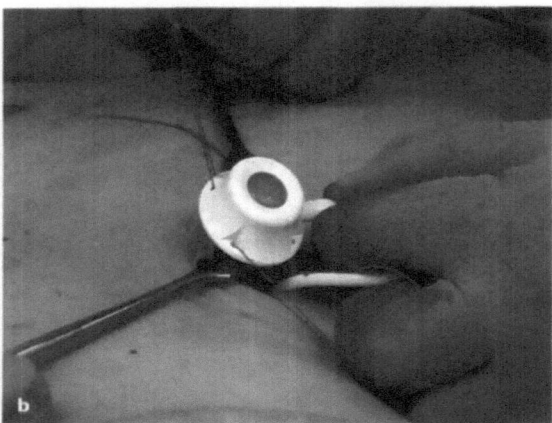

Fig. 6.8a,b. Placement of the injection port

12. *Placement of the injection port:* The trocar in the left upper quadrant is removed and the pneumoperitoneum deflated. The tubing of the silicone band is cut to an adequate length distal to the rubber-shod clamps. The tubing is connected to the saline-filled injection port with a metal connector, which is secured with two nonabsorbable ligatures (2–o) (Fig. 6.8a). The rubber-shod clamps are then removed. The self-sealing injection port is placed (with its convex side up) on the fascial sheath of the left-sided rectus muscle. To avoid migration or rotation of the injection port, it·is fixed with at least two fascial retention sutures which have to be placed in advance of final placement of the port (Fig. 6.8b). All trocars are now removed and the wounds are sutured.

13. *Adjustment of the silicone band:* According to the patient's response to the laparoscopic gastric banding, the stoma size can be adjusted by withdrawal or addition of sterile saline solution via the injection port system. This acts to deflate or inflate the inflatable balloon of the gastric band with direct influence on the stoma diameter. A change of 0.4 ml in filling volume corresponds to a change of 0.5 mm in stoma diameter. Be aware of the fact that stoma size might be temporarily decreased by stomal edema during the·early postoperative phase.

Complications

1. *Total operative mortality* is less than 1%.

2. *Stomach perforation:* The risk of perforating the stomach during dissection and tunnelization of the retrogastric area is up to 0.5%. Therefore, visual control is obligatory throughout retrogastric dissection. This is achievable, with step-by-step preparation, by pulling the already dissected posterior gastric wall ventrally. Moreover, the special snap-off splaying instrument (HOURLAY Autostatic Retractor, Duchateau, Rouvreux, Belgium) can be used for safer blunt dissection (also used for dissection of the retroesophageal window during laparoscopic fundoplication).
An important step is to fill the retrogastric tunnel with saline solution and watch out for air bubbles while insufflating air via the patient's nasal tube before the silicone band is introduced and placed around the stomach. If the retrogastric tunnel created is too narrow, band

placement with forceful drawing through the retrogastric tunnel can cause stomach perforation.

In the case of suspected gastric damage, we prefer intraoperative gastroscopy. Intragastral application of methylene blue or air insufflation into the stomach are less sensitive because a potential perforation site could be temporarily closed by the silicone band itself, which is easily recognized by endoscopy.

> ## Warning
>
> In the early postoperative period, gastric perforation has to be suspected if the patient complains of abnormal abdominal pain or shows respiratory problems (in the worst case, the patient can not be weaned off the respirator!)
>
> A gastrografin control is not always helpful because it may be false negative. Only gastroscopy is able to exclude a suspected perforation as the silicone band is clearly visible intraluminally when the gastric wall has been perforated.

3. *Pouch dilatation (up to 5%):* Incorrect placement of the silicone band, or dietary mistakes ("too much, too fast") during postoperative recovery, are most often responsible for the development of postoperative pouch dilatation. The application of a nasogastric tube into the pouch commonly relieves the symptoms and results in a reduction in pouch size.

4. *Stoma occlusion (up to 3%):* In most cases, dietary mistakes (again, "too much, too fast"; fiber-rich nutrition) are responsible. Therefore, intensive dietary instruction prior to surgery is necessary for gastric banding patients.

5. *Slippage (up to 8%):* Inadequate retention suturing is the most common cause of slippage of the gastric band. In consequence, dislocation of the silicone band to the proximal or distal stomach is possible. Aboral sections of the stomach could also dislocate in a kind of "upside-down stomach" when gastric band slippage occurs. Moreover, slippage could be caused by fulminant vomiting (following dietary mistakes), tearing the retention sutures. As a rule, laparoscopic revision should be performed.

In former series, slippage was often caused by performing the posterior dissection through the lesser sac which left the posterior wall free to move up and down. Therefore, the retrogastric dissection plane should be clearly above the peritoneal reflection of the bursa omentalis.

6. *Gastric wall erosion by the silicone band (up to 2%):* To a great extent, erosion of the stomach wall caused by the implanted gastric band is clinically inapparent, but could also provoke severe symptoms such as gastric bleeding. Laparoscopy (or laparotomy), with removal of the band and suturing of the lesion, is indispensable.

7. *Pulmonary embolism, wound infection (1% – 2%):* Obese patients have an increased incidence of risk factors for coronary heart disease such as hyperlipidemia, hypertension, and type II diabetes mellitus. Intensive peri- and postoperative care and control reduces the complication rate.

8. *Complications of the injection port (up to 5%):* Migration or rotation of the injection port can occur when fixation of the port on the fascial sheath of the rectus muscle is (or has become) inadequate. Accessing the port chamber with an inappropriate needle could cause port leakage and may require surgical replacement of the port. Prior to accessing the port, and while positioning the injection needle, the port should be located by ultrasonography (or radiologically for the port being radiopaque) to avoid injection into the tissue or even damage to the port connecting tube.

9. *Conversion rate (3%):* Be aware of a learning curve.

Overall Results

1. Substantial weight loss generally occurs within 12 months following surgery (up to 60% of excess weight). Some weight is regained within 2 – 5 years.
2. With weight loss comes improvement in the co-morbid conditions that often accompany obesity.

Bibliography

Balsiger BM, de Leon EL, Sarr MG (1997) Surgical treatment of obesity: who is an appropriate candidate? Mayo Clin Proc 72:551–558

Belachew M, Legrand M, Vincent V, Lismonde M, Ledocte N, Deschamps V (1998) Laparoscopic adjustable gastric banding. World J Surg 22:955–963

Benotti PN, Forse RA (1995) The role of gastric surgery in the multidisciplinary management of severe obesity. Am J Surg 169:361–367

Kunath U, Menari B (1995) Laparoskopisches "gastric banding" zur Behandlung der pathologischen Adipositas. Chirurg 66:1263–1267

Kuzmak L, Burak E (1993) Pouch enlargement: myth or reality? Impressions from serial upper gastrointestinal series in silicone gastric banding patients. Obes Surg 3:57–62

Kuzmak L, Ricker R (1991) Pathologic changes in the stomach at the site of silicone gastric banding. Obes Surg 1:63–86

Peterli R, Strub R, Herzig U, Ackermann Ch, Schuppisser IP, Tondelli P (1999) Steigende Frequenz bariatrisch-chirurgischer Eingriffe seit Ersatz der Gastroplastik durch das laparoskopische Magenband zur Behandlung der morbiden Adipositas. Chirurg 70:190–195

Pier A, Abtaki G, Lipper H (1999) Chirurgische Therapie der pathologischen Adipositas durch laparoskopisches "gastric banding". Chirurg 70:196–205

Sagar PM (1995) Surgical treatment of morbid obesity. Br J Surg 82:732–739

Weiner R, Emmerlich V, Wasner D, Bockhorn H (1998) Management und Therapie von postoperativen Komplikationen nach "gastric banding" wegen morbider Adipositas. Chirurg 69:1082–1088

Totally Laparoscopic Distal Gastrectomy with Extended Lymph Node Dissection

I. Uyama, A. Sugioka, J. Fujita, and A. Hasumi

Since the first laparoscopic gastrectomy was performed in 1992 on a patient with gastric ulcer (Goh et al. 1992), several authors have documented the cases of laparoscopic gastrectomy not only for gastric ulcer, but also for gastric cancer (Kuo et al. 1998; Nagai et al. 1995; Kitano et al. 1995; Uyama et al. 1995; Mayers and Orebaugh 1998; Carios et al. 1996). However, the procedure of totally laparoscopic gastrectomy with extended lymph node dissection has not been established. Herein, we describe our procedure of totally laparoscopic distal gastrectomy with D2 extraperigastric lymph node dissection.

Definition of Regional Lymph Nodes of the Stomach

As shown in Fig. 7.1, the numbers and groups of the regional lymph nodes are defined according to the general rules of the Japanese Research Society for Gastric Cancer (1995). We routinely apply D2 lymph node dissection, in which both group 1 and 2 lymph nodes were dissected, for the patients with early gastric cancer located in the middle or lower third of the stomach. Group 1 lymph nodes consisted of right cardial lymph nodes (No. 1), lymph nodes along the lesser curvature (No. 3), lymph nodes along the left gastroepiploic vessels (No. 4sb), lymph nodes along the right gastroepiploic vessels (No. 4d), suprapyloric lymph nodes (No. 5), and infrapyloric lymph nodes (No. 6). Group 2 consisted of lymph nodes along the left gastric artery (No. 7), lymph nodes along the common hepatic artery (No. 8a), lymph nodes around the celiac artery (No. 9), and lymph nodes along the splenic artery (No. 11).

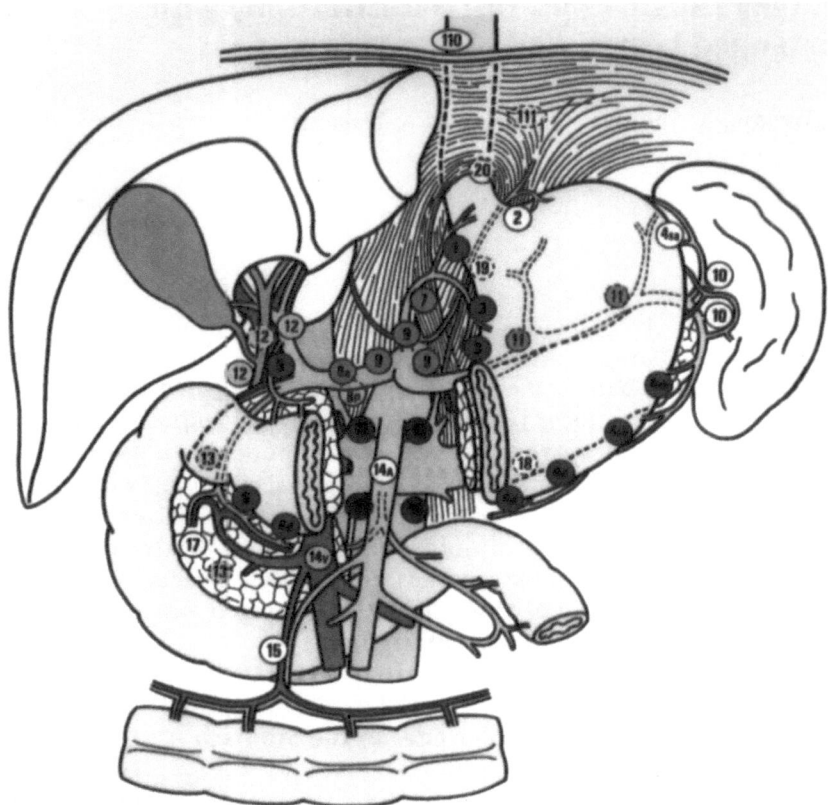

Fig. 7.1. Lymph node station numbers. In D2 lymph node dissection, group 1 and 2 lymph nodes are dissected. *Red circles*, group 1; *blue circles*, group 2

Patient Selection and Preoperative Preparation

Indications for laparoscopic distal gastrectomy were as follows: (a) The tumor was located in the middle or lower third of the stomach; (b) the depth of tumoral invasion was confined to the submucosal layer (T1); (c) lymph node metastasis was not evident (N0) or confined to group 1 (N1); (d) the tumor was not suitable for either endoscopic mucosal resection or (laparoscopic) local resection. Tumor size and histologic types were not included to the criteria. Patients with unfavorable medical conditions for general anesthesia were excluded. A history of upper abdominal surgery was not necessarily a contraindication. In this series, seven patients were enrolled, six with early gastric cancer and one with malignant lymphoma

Preoperatively, 400 ml of autologous blood were stored. For easy identification of a lesion during operation, each lesion was endoscopically marked with four clips (MD-59; Olympus Optical, Tokyo, Japan) using a clip applicator (HX-4 U; Olympus Optical) and stained with 0.5 ml an indian ink.

Operating-Room and Patient Set-Up

Under general anesthesia, the patients were placed in a supine position with legs apart in a 20° reverse Trendelenburg position. The operator stood to the patient's right side, while the first assistant stood to the left and the camera operator between the patient's legs. Two video monitors were placed over the patient's shoulders.

Surgical Techniques

Five to six ports, 12 mm in diameter, were placed as shown in Fig. 7.2. Pneumoperitoneum was established using an open technique. The flexible electrolaparoscope (Fujinon Corporation, Tokyo, Japan), indispens-

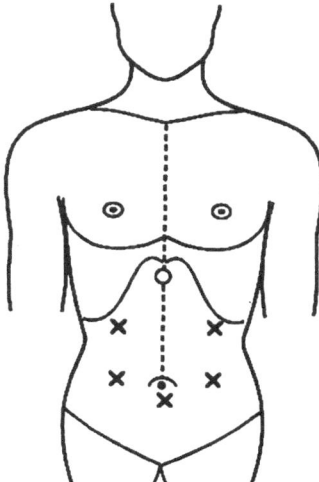

Fig. 7.2. Port positions. *Crosses*, standard ports; *open circle*, optional port. The ports are all 12 mm in size. Infraumbilical port for camera operator; right midclavicular ports for the operator; left midclavicular ports for first assistant; subxiphoid port for hepatic retractor

able for this procedure, was introduced through the port in the infraumbilicus. Localization of a lesion could be roughly identified extraluminally as an area stained with indian ink.

Lymph Node Dissection Along the Right and Left Gastroepiploic Vessels

The procedure was started with the dissection of Nos. 4d and 4sb lymph nodes, dividing the gastrocolic ligament proximally about 4 cm apart from the epiploic arcade, towards the lower pole of the spleen, using laparosonic coagulating shears(LCS; Ethicon, Cincinnati, OH). The roots of the left gastroepiploic vessels were exposed using a laparoscopic ultrasonic surgical dissector (LUSA) and divided with double clips (Fig. 7.3a).

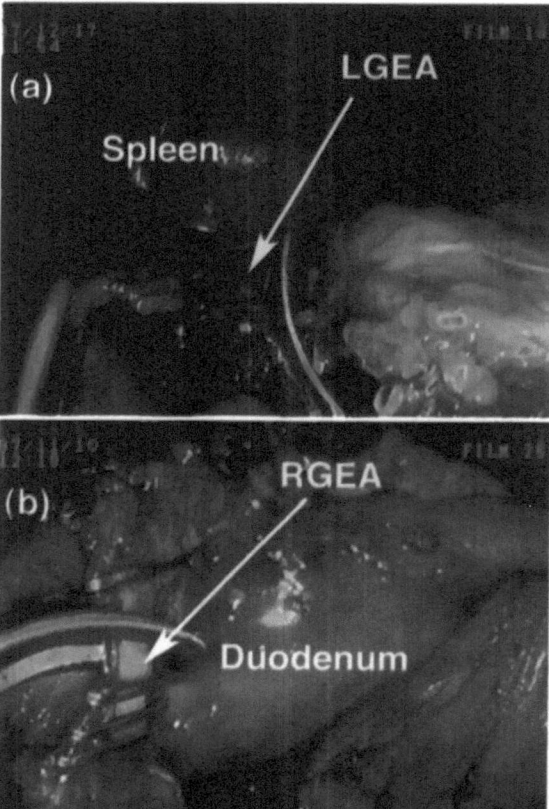

Fig. 7.3a–b. a Exposure and division of the left gastroepiploic artery. **b** Exposure and division of the right gastroepiploic artery. *LGEA*, left gastroepiploic artery; *RGEA*, right gastroepiploic artery

Infrapyloric and Suprapyloric Lymph Node Dissection

The division of the gastrocolic ligament was advanced distally towards the pyloric ring using LCS. The roots of the right gastroepiploic vessels were exposed using LUSA and divided with double clips (Fig. 7.3b). The No. 6 lymph nodes were dissected from the duodenum using LCS. The root of the right gastric artery was exposed using LUSA and divided with double clips (Fig. 7.4a). The No. 5 lymph nodes, along with the right gastric artery, were dissected from the lesser curvature using LCS. The duodenum was resected 1 cm distally from the pyloric ring using an endoscopic stapling device.

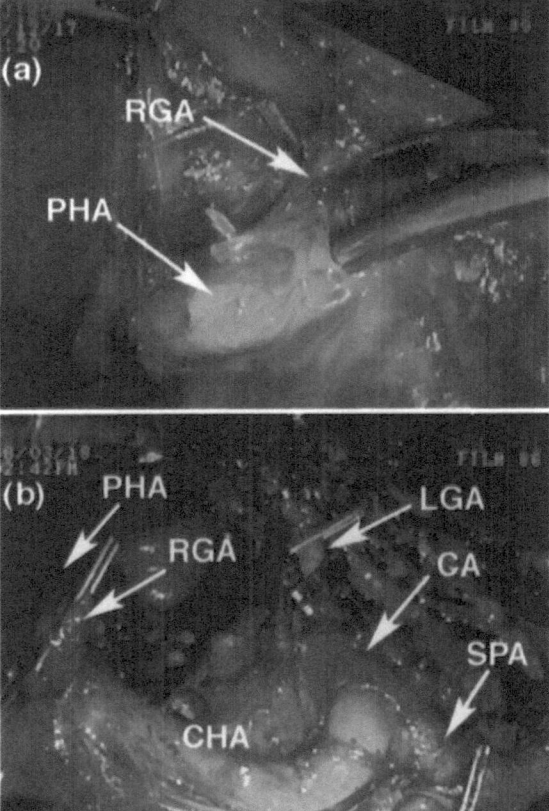

Fig. 7.4a – b. a Exposure and division of the right gastric artery. **b** Dissection of Nos. 7, 8a, 9, and 11 lymph nodes. *PHA*, proper hepatic artery; *RGA*, stump of right gastric artery; *LGA*, left gastric artery; *CA*, celiac artery; *SPA*, splenic artery; *CHA*, common hepatic artery

Lymph Node Dissection Along the Common Hepatic, Celiac, Splenic, and Left Gastric Arteries

Caudal retraction of the pancreas with the Endoretractor II (United States Surgical Corporation, Norwalk, CT, USA) facilitated exposure of the common hepatic, splenic, and celiac arteries (Nos. 8a, 9, and 11, respectively), and lymph node dissection along with each artery using LUSA and LCS (Fig. 7.4b). The left gastric vein was divided. The root of the left gastric artery was exposed and divided with double clips, which enabled dissection of the No. 7 lymph node (Fig. 7.4b).

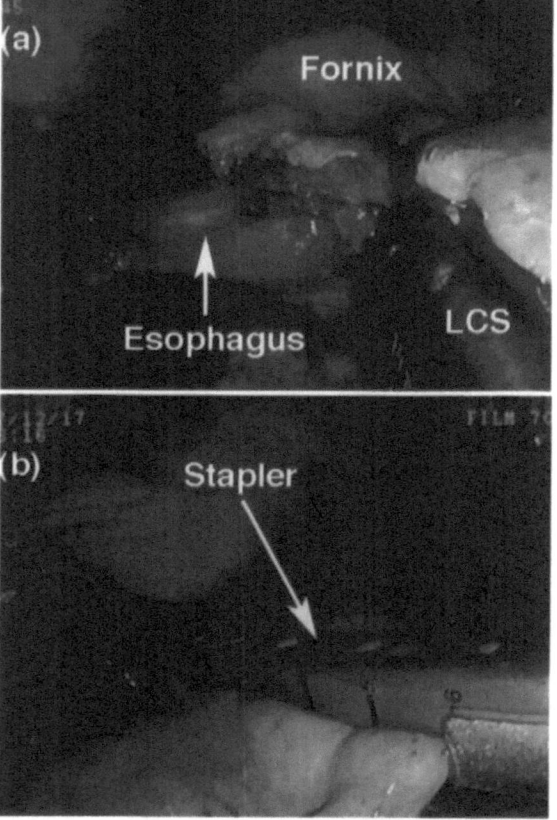

Fig. 7.5a-b. a Dissection of the No. 1 lymph nodes along with skeletonization of the upper third of the lesser curvature. *LCS*, laparosonic coagulating shears. **b** Transection of the stomach using stapler

Right Cardial Lymph Node Dissection and Transection of the Stomach

The right cardial lymph node (No. 1) was dissected along with skeletonization of the upper third of the lesser curvature (Fig. 7.5a). The resection line was finally determined using the intraoperative gastroendoscopy, confirming the location of the tumor with the intragastric clips applied preoperatively. The stomach was transected using an endoscopic stapling device (Fig. 7.5b). The resected stomach was set aside in a plastic specimen bag (Endocatch II; United States Surgical Corporation, Norwalk, CT, USA) and placed in the right subphrenic space or in the pelvic cavity temporarily.

Reconstruction

An intracorporeal Roux-en-Y gastrojejunostomy was applied for reconstruction. The transverse colon was retracted cephalad to expose the ligament of Treitz, and the jejunum was divided 20 cm distal of the ligament using an endoscopic stapling device. The jejunal loop was pulled up to near the gastric remnant in an antecolic manner. The gastrojejunostomy was created with a functional end-to-end anastomosis using an endoscopic stapling device. Both corners of the jejunal loop and the gastric remnant were excised to make holes, and each jaw of the endoscopic stapling device, which was introduced through the left upper port, was passed into the lumina through both holes. The jaws were closed and the device activated, converting the two holes into one common hole. These procedures were repeated between two and three times until a sufficient anastomotic lumen was obtained. The common hole was closed using two or three stapling devices.

Jejunojejunostomy was made 50 cm distal of the gastrojejunostomy site using the same stapling technique. The mesenteric gap was repaired with hernia staplers. The accomplished Roux-en-Y reconstruction is shown in Fig. 7.6.

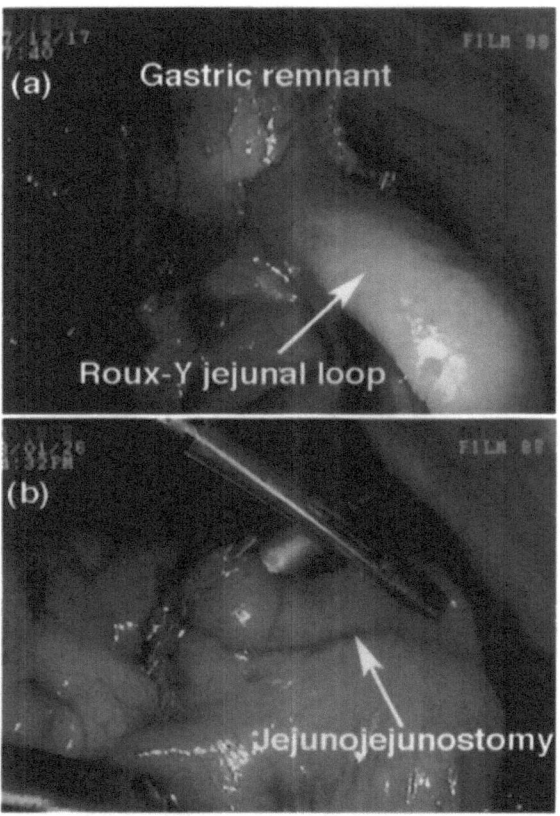

Fig. 7.6a,b. Completed Roux-en-Y reconstruction. **a** Gastrojejunostomy using the functional end-to-end anastomotic technique. **b** Jejunojejunostomy

Removal of the Resected Stomach

The right lower trocar wound was extended to approximately 3.5 cm and the plastic specimen bag containing the resected stomach was removed. Two drains were placed through the bilateral trocar wound and the whole procedure was completed with wound closure (Fig. 7.7).

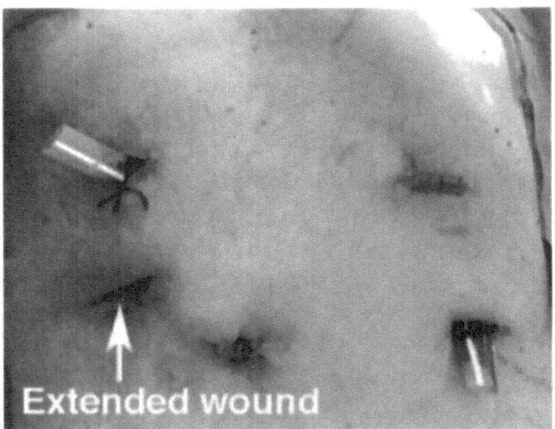

Fig. 7.7. The operative wound

Current Results

We have performed totally laparoscopic distal gastrectomy with D2 extraperigastric lymph node dissection in seven patients, six with early gastric cancer and one with malignant lymphoma.

In all patients, totally laparoscopic procedures were completed without any conversion to open surgery. There was no mortality in this series. One patient experienced an anastomotic stricture, which was resolved with endoscopic balloon dilatation, and another patient suffered from Roux-en-Y stasis syndrome, constituting a morbidity rate of 28.6%.

The mean operating time was 487.6 min (range, 389–454 min), which was significantly longer compared to open surgery (data not shown). The mean blood loss was 246.2 ml (range, 56–454 ml) and no blood transfusion other than autologous blood was required. All surgical margins were free from cancer cells and the mean number of dissected lymph nodes per patient was 45.2 (range, 25–74), which was statistically the same as that of open surgery. The mean day of initial postoperative mobility (walking) (1.8 days; range, 1–3 days) and commencement on a liquid diet (4.2 days; range, 3–7 days) were sooner and the mean sum total use times of analgesics (2.1 times; range 0–3) fewer compared with open surgery.

Conclusions

These results indicated that laparoscopic distal gastrectomy with extended lymph node dissection for early gastric cancer and malignant lymphoma afforded the same degree of safety and curability as open surgery, while the less invasive nature of the approach can be considered an unequivocal advantage of laparoscopy. We have also successfully performed totally laparoscopic total gastrectomy and proximal gastrectomy. It is expected that these procedures of totally laparoscopic gastrectomy with extended lymph node dissection would reasonably be applied to further advanced cases and become standard procedures for gastric malignancies.

References

Carios BL, Xavier BV, Marco C, Mato R, Ruggiero R (1996) Laparoscopic Billroth II distal subtotal gastrectomy with gastric stump suspension for gastric malignancies. Am J Surg 171(2):289–292

Goh P, Tekant Y, Isaac J, Kum CK, Ngoi SS (1992) The technique of laparoscopic Billroth II gastrectomy. Surg Laparosc Endosc 2(3):258–260

Japanese Research Society for Gastric Cancer (1995) Japanese classification of gasrtic carcinoma, first English edition. Kanehara & Co., Tokyo, pp. 4–35

Kitano S, Shimoda K, Miyahara M, Shiraishi N, Bandoh T, Yoshida T, Shuto K, Kobayashi M (1995) Laparoscopic approaches in the management of patients with early gastric carcinomas. Surg Laparosc Endosc 5(5):359–362

Kuo WH, Lee WJ, Chen CN, Yuan RH, Yu SC (1998) Laparoscopic subtotal gastrectomy with lymphadenectomy in a patient with early gastric cancer. J Formos Med Assoc 97(2):127–130

Mayers TM, Orebaugh MG (1998) Totally laparoscopic Billroth I gastrectomy. J Am Coll Surg 186(l):100–103

Nagai Y, Tanimura H, Takifuji K, Kashiwagi H, Yamoto H, Nakatani Y (1995) Laparoscope-assisted Billroth I gastrectomy. Surg Laparosc Endosc 5(4):281–287

Uyama I, Ogiwara H, Takahara T, Furuta T, Kikuchi K, Iida S (1995) Laparoscopic minilaparotomy Billroth I gastrectomy with extraperigastric lymphadenectomy for early gastric cancer using an abdominal wall-lifting method. J Laparoendosc Surg 5(3): 181–187

Laparoscopic Surgery for Early Gastric Cancer: Lesion-Lifting Method and Intragastric Mucosal Resection

M. Ohgami, Y. Otani, T. Furukawa, K. Kumai, T. Kubota, J. Tokuyama, Y.-I. Kim, and M. Kitajima

Background

Asymptomatic early gastric cancers, especially lesions in which infiltration is limited to the mucosa, have frequently been detected through a well-established screening program in Japan (Hisamichi and Sugawara 1984; Hiki 1991). The accuracy of preoperative diagnosis of the depth of cancerous infiltration for mucosal gastric cancer is as high as 79% – 90% by endoscopy and endoscopic ultrasonography (Kida et al. 1993; Fujisaki et al. 1993). Therefore, it is important to establish minimally invasive therapy for mucosal gastric cancer. Among 473 consecutive patients with mucosal gastric cancers who underwent gastrectomies with lymph node dissection at our institution, lymph node metastasis was found in

Table 8.1. Lymph node metastasis in mucosal gastric cancer[a]

Macroscopic type	Number (–)	Number (+)	Total
Elevated type (IIa)	67 (100%)	0 (0%)	67 (100%)
Depressive type (IIc)	370 (97.6%)	9 (2.4%)	379 (100%)
Mixed type	26 (96.3%)	1[b] (3.7%)	27 (100%)
Total	463 (97.9%)	10[c] (2.1%)	473 (100%)

[a] Histologic results of patients with mucosal gastric cancer who underwent gastrectomies with systematic lymph node dissection in Keio University Hospital between 1964 and 1999.
[b] IIa+IIc.
[c] The cases with lymph node metastasis had mostly ulcer and relatively large lesions (39±15 mm) with poorly differentiated adenocarcinoma.

only ten patients (2.1%), most of whom had large depressed lesions with ulcer or scar formation (Otani et al. 1995) (Table 8.1). However, there was no lymph node metastasis when the diameter of the lesion was less than 25 mm. Therefore, the majority of mucosal gastric cancers can be curatively treated by local resection of stomach tissue. In order to obtain both complete cure and minimal invasiveness, we introduced two different laparoscopic procedures, chosen according to the site of the lesion, in March 1992. One is laparoscopic wedge resection of the stomach using a lesion-lifting method, and the other is laparoscopic intragastric mucosal resection.

Indications

Indications for these two laparoscopic procedures are as follows:

1. The lesion is preoperatively diagnosed as mucosal cancer.
2. Diameter is < 25 mm, if the lesion is the elevated type.
3. Diameter is < 15 mm and there is no ulcer formation if the lesion is the depressed type.
4. The lesion-lifting method is applied for lesions of the anterior wall, the lesser curvature, and the greater curvature of the stomach with a sufficient distance from the cardia and pylorus, while laparoscopic intragastric mucosal resection is applied for lesions of the posterior wall of the stomach and lesions near the cardia or the pylorus.
   According to the result of final histology of the resected specimen, curability of the surgery is evaluated. Our criteria of histologic findings which lead to additional open gastrectomy with lymph node dissection include: (1) Positive surgical margin, (2) positive venous or lymphatic cancer invasion, or (3) cancer infiltration into the middle or deep portion of the submucosal layer (> sm2) (Kurihara et al. 1998).

Procedures

Laparoscopic Wedge Resection of the Stomach Using a Lesion-Lifting Method

The lesion-lifting method (Ohgami et al. 1994a,b, 1999) comprises the placement of marking clips around the cancerous lesion during preoperative gastroscopy to localize the lesion during surgery, and the sites of the marking clips are confirmed to be cancer-negative by biopsies

(Fig. 8.1). This procedure is important not only for easy localization of the lesion during surgery, but also to ensure a sufficient surgical margin.

The entire surgical procedure is performed laparoscopically under general anesthesia. An initial trocar for a laparoscope is inserted at the umbilicus using Hasson's technique, and pneumoperitoneum is created with carbon dioxide. Three additional trocars are inserted in the upper abdomen (Fig. 8.2). The abdominal cavity is fully investigated, and the location of the cancerous lesion is confirmed with the assistance of intraoperative gastroscopy. When the lesion is located on the greater

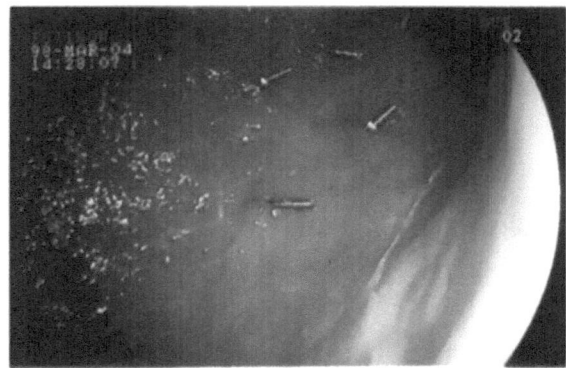

Fig. 8.1. Marking clips are placed around the cancerous lesion during preoperative gastroscopy to localize the lesion during surgery, and the sites of the marking clips are confirmed to be cancer-negative by biopsies

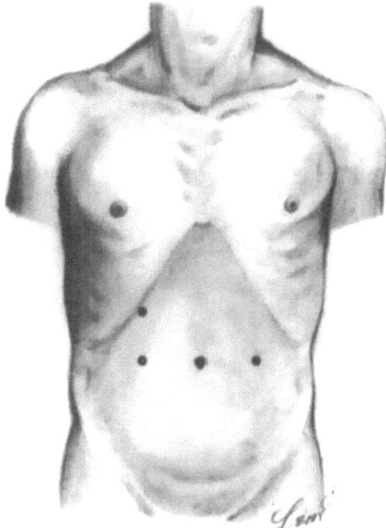

Fig. 8.2. Trocar placement in the laparoscopic wedge resection using a lesion-lifting method. An initial trocar for a laparoscope is inserted at the umbilicus using Hasson's technique, and three additional trocars are inserted in the upper abdomen

curvature or the lesser curvature of the stomach, the gastric wall surrounding the lesion is devascularized and exposed using an ultrasonic dividing device (Laparosonic Coagulating Shears; Ethicon Endo-Surgery, New Brunswick, NJ, USA) in advance. After exposure, the gastric wall near the lesion is grasped and lifted towards the abdominal wall by atraumatic forceps. The abdominal wall above the lesion and the gastric wall in the vicinity of the lesion is pierced by a 12-G sheathed needle (Fig. 8.3). The needle is removed, and the outer sheath is left in place. A small metal rod with a fine wire at the center is introduced through the outer sheath into the stomach (Fig. 8.4), and the outer sheath is removed. Finally, by pulling the wire, the lesion is lifted precisely by the

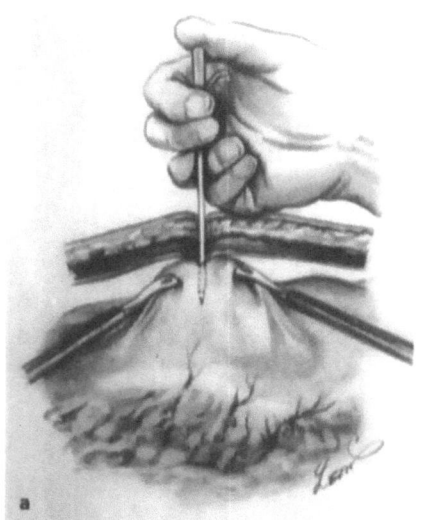

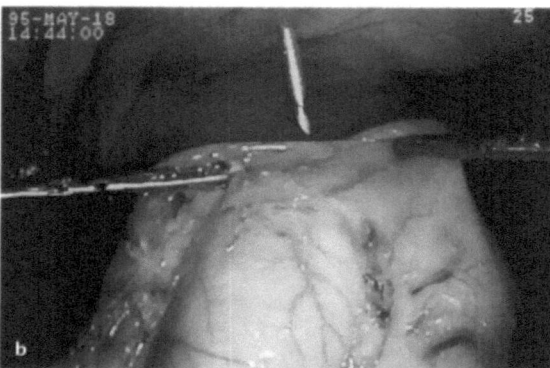

Figs. 8.3a,b. After complete exposure of the gastric wall around the lesion, the gastric wall near the lesion is grasped and lifted towards the abdominal wall by atraumatic forceps. The abdominal wall above the lesion and the gastric wall in the vicinity of the lesion is pierced by a 12-G sheathed needle

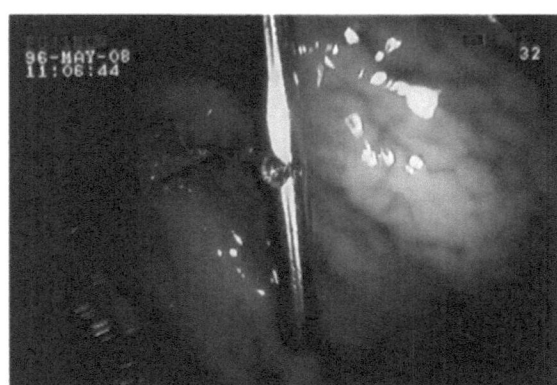

Fig. 8.4. A small metal rod with a fine wire at the center is introduced through the outer sheath into the stomach

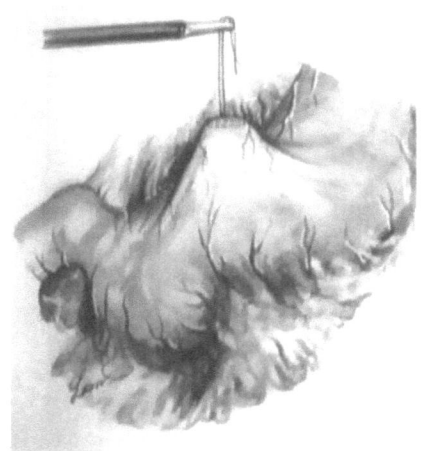

Fig. 8.5. The lesion is lifted precisely by the metal rod by pulling the wire

metal rod (Fig. 8.5). Wedge resection is performed using a multifire endoscopic stapling device, allowing a sufficient distance from the metal rod (Fig. 8.6). Between three and five staple cartridges are usually required for the resection. During the procedure, a gastroscope is kept in place in the stomach as a stent in order to avoid stenosis or severe deformity. The resected specimen is isolated within a specimen bag (Fig. 8.7), and retrieved from the umbilical wound. Perigastric lymph nodes along the greater curvature are resected in some cases for sampling in patients in whom submucosal cancer infiltration cannot be completely ruled out. When the lesser omentum or the greater omentum is opened, it is closed using hernia staples. Hemostasis along the staple line is confirmed lapa-

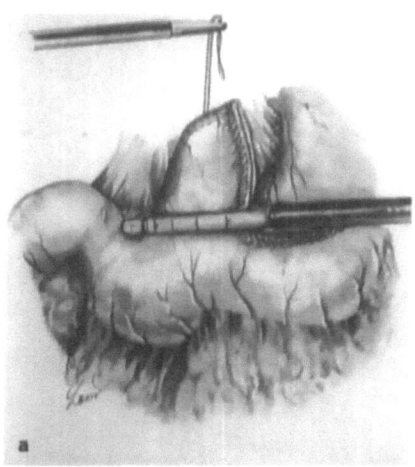

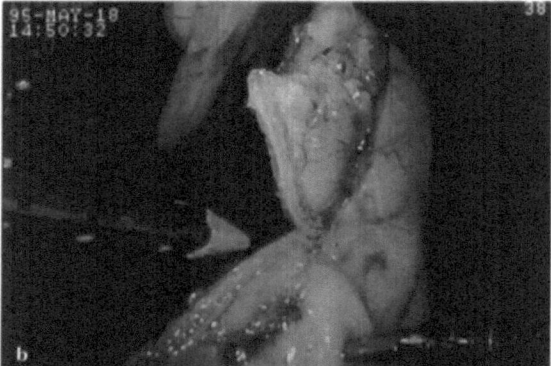

Figs. 8.6a,b. Wedge resection is performed using a multifire endoscopic stapling device, allowing a sufficient distance from the metal rod. Between three and five staple cartridges are usually required for the resection

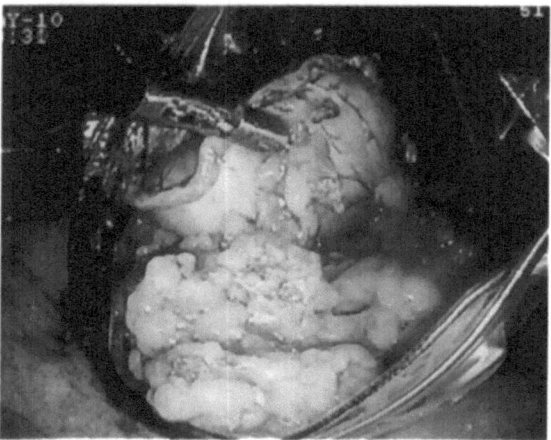

Fig. 8.7. The resected specimen is isolated within a specimen bag and retrieved from the umbilical wound

roscopically and gastroscopically. Trocar wounds are cosmetically closed and the operation is completed.

If the resected specimen has all of the preoperatively placed marking clips, it automatically suggests that there is a sufficient surgical margin, because the preoperative biopsies have given cancer-negative results at the sites of marking clips. Perigastric lymph nodes along the greater curvature of the stomach can be also resected for sampling, if necessary (Fig. 8.8). Full thickness specimen is obtained, therefore, detailed histologic examination can be achieved (Fig. 8.9). Histologic results in our series for 6 years from 1992 are shown in Table 8.2.

Operative scarring is minimal (Fig. 8.10), and postoperative pain is negligible. Patients can start on a liquid diet within 1–2 days following surgery, and they can usually be discharged within 5 days.

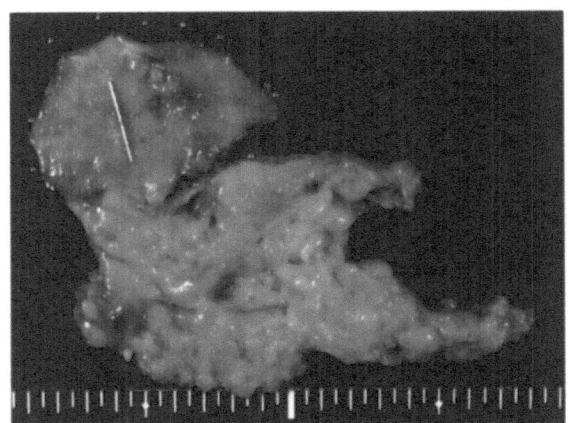

Fig. 8.8. A full-thickness specimen is obtained and perigastric lymph nodes can also be resected for sampling, if necessary

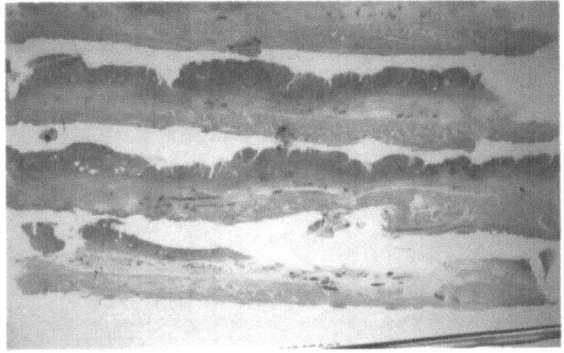

Fig. 8.9. Detailed histologic examination can be achieved

Table 8.2. Histologic results in lesion-lifting method and laparoscopic intragastric mucosal resection (LIM) in our 6 years experience from 1992

	Lesion-lifting method (*n*=79)	LIM (*n*=18)
Lesion size (mm)	5±7 (5–30)	9±6 (5–25)
Specimen size (mm)	67±13 (50–110)	48±8 (42–65)
Surgical margin (mm)	15±6 (6–30)	8±4 (2–15)
Macroscopic type	Protruded (type I): 2 Elevated (type IIa): 23 Flat (type IIb): 1 Depressed (type IIc): 52 Mixed (type IIc+IIa): 1	Elevated (type IIa): 3 Depressed (type IIc): 15
Histologic type[a]	Well: 56; mod: 11; poor: 6 sig: 6	Well: 17; mod: 1
Cancer infiltration[b]	m: 70; sm1: 8; sm2: 1[c]	m: 17; sm1: 1
Lymphatic or venous invasion	Negative: 77; positive: 2[c]	Negative: 18

[a] Well, well differentiated adenocarcinoma; mod, moderately differentiated adenocarcinoma; poor, poorly differentiated adenocarcinoma; sig, signet-ring cell carcinoma.
[b] m, Mucosal cancer. Submucosal infiltration depth is divided into three categories, sm1, sm2, and sm3, by dividing the submucosal layer into three equal parts.
[c] Three cases with sm2 cancer infiltration or positive lymphatic invasion underwent open gastrectomies with systematic lymph node dissection 4 weeks after intial laparoscopic surgery. However, there were no residual cancer cells on histology.

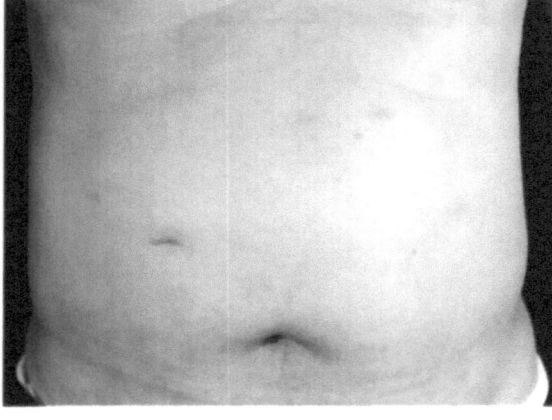

Fig. 8.10. Operative scarring is minimal with the lesion-lifting method

Laparoscopic Intragastric Mucosal Resection

Laparoscopic intragastric mucosal resection (Ohashi 1995; Ohgami and Kitajima 1995; Ohgami et al. 1999) consists in marking the cancerous lesion with marking clips preoperatively, and intraoperative gastroscopy is used as in the lesion-lifting method. An initial trocar for a laparoscope is inserted at the umbilicus using Hasson's technique, and pneumoperitoneum is created with carbon dioxide. Two additional trocars are inserted in the upper abdomen (Fig. 8.11). The abdominal cavity is fully investigated, and the location of the cancerous lesion is confirmed by gastroscopy. After the duodenal bulb is occluded with a bowel clamp, the stomach is insufflated via the gastroscope. The abdominal wall and the anterior wall of the stomach are pierced with three balloon trocars (Marlow Surgical Technologies, Willoughby, OH, USA) laparoscopically and gastroscopically (Fig. 8.12). The tips of the trocars are placed in the

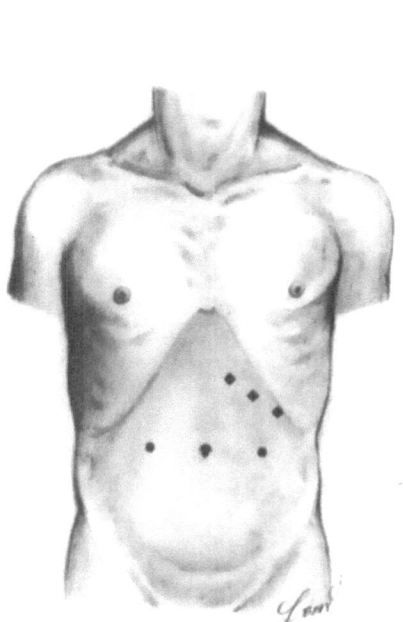

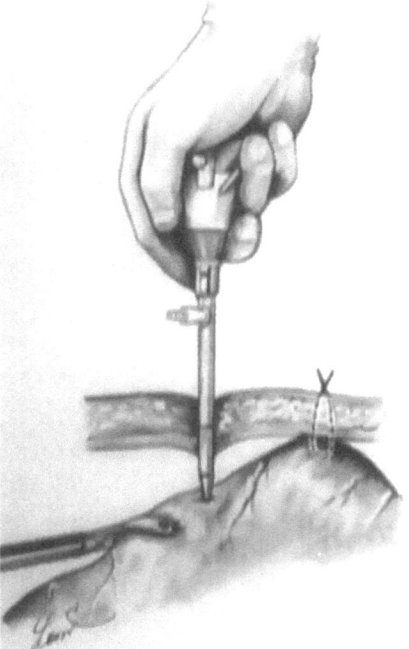

Fig. 8.11. Trocar placement in laparoscopic intragastric mucosal resection. Circles, usual trocar; diamonds, balloon trocar

Fig. 8.12. The abdominal wall and the anterior wall are pierced with three balloon trocars laparoscopically and gastroscopically

stomach and their balloons are inflated to secure the trocars. Pneumoperitoneum is then evacuated, and the stomach is insufflated with carbon dioxide through a balloon trocar, maintaining a maximum pressure
of 10 mmHg. A thin, rigid scope (5 mm) is introduced into the stomach
through the central balloon trocar, and operative instruments are introduced into the stomach through the others (intragastric surgery)
(Figs. 8.13, 8.14). The lesion is confirmed and the margin of resection is
marked by electrocautery, allowing a sufficient surgical margin. Physiologic saline solution with dilute adrenaline (0.01%) is injected into the

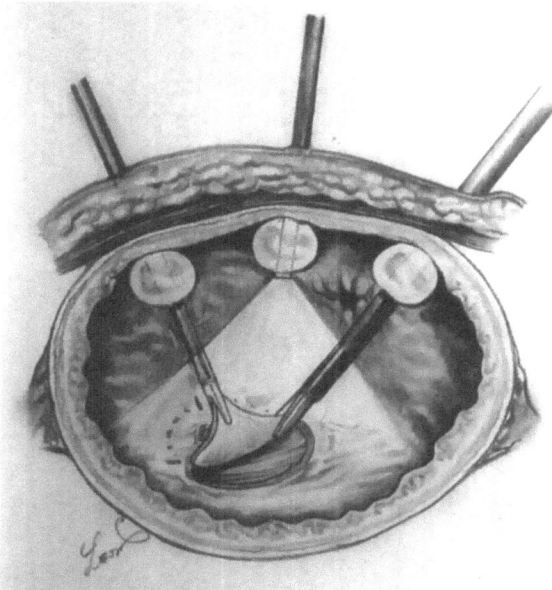

Fig. 8.13. A thin, rigid
scope (5 mm) is intro-
duced into the stomach
through the central bal-
loon trocar, and operative
instruments are intro-
duced into the stomach
through the other trocars
(intragastric surgery)

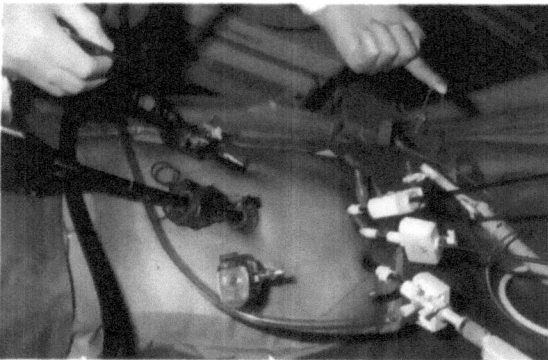

Fig. 8.14. Appearance of
trocar placement in intragastric surgery

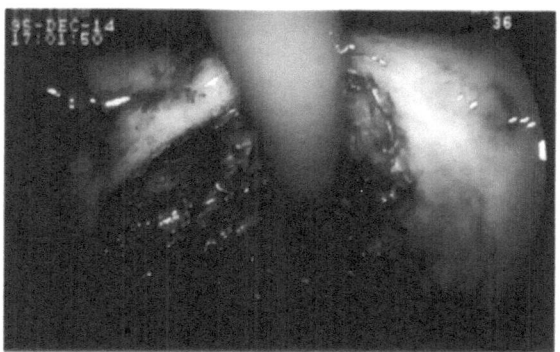

Fig. 8.15. The margin of resection is marked by electrocautery, allowing a sufficient surgical margin. The mucosal and submucosal layer of the marked area is dissected and resected using electrocautery or an ultrasonic dividing device, leaving the muscle layer intact

submucosal layer under the resected area to obtain easy exposure of the plane of dissection and to reduce bleeding during dissection. The mucosal and submucosal layer of the marked area is dissected and resected using electrocautery or an ultrasonic dividing device, leaving the muscle layer intact (Fig. 8.15). The resected specimen is isolated in a specimen bag and retrieved by a gastroscope via the mouth. Hemostasis in the area of resection is confirmed, and the balloon trocars are removed from the stomach. Pneumoperitoneum is again created and the trocar holes of the stomach are closed. Trocar wounds are cosmetically closed and the operation is completed.

In a resected specimen, a sufficient distance from the lesion to any surgical margin can be obtained (Figs. 8.16, 8.17). Histologic results in our series for six years from 1992 are shown in Table 8.2.

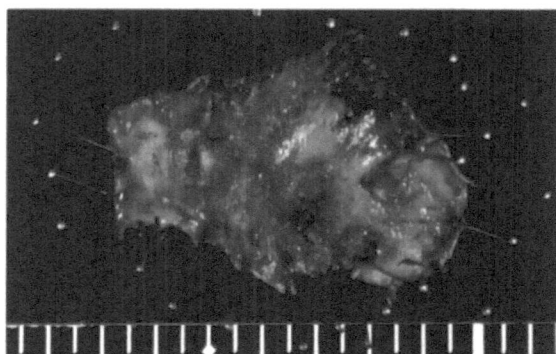

Fig. 8.16. There is a sufficient surgical margin in the resected specimen

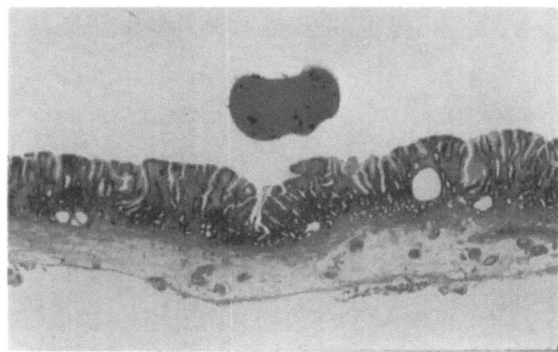

Fig. 8.17. Histology revealed that cancer infiltration was limited within the mucosal layer and there was a sufficient surgical margin horizontally and vertically

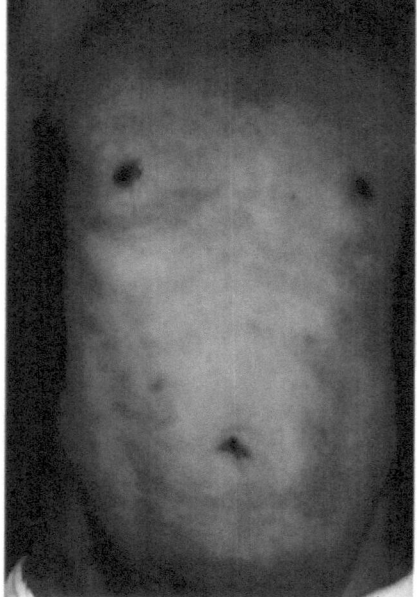

Fig. 8.18. Operative scarring is minimal in laparoscopic intragastric mucosal resection

Operative scarring is minimal (Fig. 8.18), and postoperative pain is negligible. Patients can start on a liquid diet within 2–3 days following surgery, and they can usually be discharged within 7–8 days.

Advantages

The advantages of these laparoscopic methods include: (1) They are minimally invasive; therefore, postoperative pain is negligible and patients can recover quickly and return to normal activity early after surgery, (2) a sufficient surgical margin can be obtained horizontally and vertically, (3) a detailed histologic examination is feasible, and (4) most of the stomach is preserved.

Problems and Pitfalls

Accuracy of preoperative diagnosis of the depth of cancer infiltration is most important in the indication for a laparoscopic procedure for early gastric cancer, because an additional open gastrectomy may be required after laparoscopic surgery due to the risk of lymph node metastasis when the infiltration is underestimated. A combination of radiographic examination, endoscopy, and endoscopic ultrasonography in preoperative diagnosis is helpful for the accuracy (Fujisaki et al. 1993; Kida et al. 1993).

Because the laparoscopic procedures described involve local excision preserving most of the stomach, there remains the problem of multicentric gastric cancer. Tada et al. (1993) reported that the possibility of either simultaneous or metachronous multicentric gastric cancer was as high as 5% – 15 %. In our series, we also experienced three cases with metachronous early gastric cancer during the follow-up period after initial laparoscopic surgery (Ohgami et al., 1999). Again, they were all found as mucosal cancer and successfully treated by open gastrectomy, laser irradiation, and endoscopic mucosal resection, respectively. During a follow-up period after laparoscopic surgery for early gastric cancer, not only the recurrence of cancer, but also metachronous gastric cancer should be carefully sought by means of periodic gastroscopy (every 6 months).

If laparoscopic intragastric mucosal resection is applied for the lesion near the cardia, it may result in stenosis in the cardia and the lower esophagus during the healing of ulcers in the resected area (Ohgami et al., 1999). Therefore, the patient should be carefully monitored by endoscopy weekly following surgery until the ulcer is completely healed. If stenosis is found in the cardia or the lower esophagus, endoscopic balloon dilatation can be used to treat the stenosis.

Recently, there have been reports about trocar site recurrence after

laparoscopic surgery for malignancy, especially after laparoscopic colorectal surgery and laparoscopic gallbladder surgery (Alexander et al.
1993; Wexner and Cohen 1995; Cirocco et al. 1994). In these reports, most
of the initial malignancies seemed to be at an advanced stage in which
the cancer extended beyond the serosa, or the gallbladder was ruptured
during surgery. Some report that pneumoperitoneum with carbon dioxide may increase the risk of tumor implantation (Jones et al. 1995; Bouvy
et al. 1996); however, its mechanism and risk in clinical practice is still
controversial and unknown (Thomas et al. 1996; Whelan et al. 1996).
Our indications for laparoscopic surgery for early gastric cancer are
strictly limited to mucosal cancer, and we cautiously isolated the
resected specimen in a specimen bag immediately after resection to
avoid the risk of implantation of cancer tissue. We have never experienced a trocar site implantation in our series.

Conclusion

If the patient is selected properly, laparoscopic wedge resection of the
stomach using a lesion-lifting method and laparoscopic intragastric
mucosal resection can be a curative and minimally invasive treatment
for early gastric cancer.

References

Alexander RJT, Jaques BC, Mitchell KG (1993) Laparoscopically assisted colectomy
  and wound recurrence. Lancet 341:249
Bouvy ND, Marquet RL, Jeekel H, Bonjer HJ (1996) Impact of gas(less) laparoscopy
  and laparotomy on peritoneal tumor growth and abdominal wall metastases. Ann
  Surg 224:694–700
Cirocco WC, Schwartzman A, Golub RW (1994) Abdominal wall recurrence after lapa-
  roscopic colectomy for colon cancer. Surgery 116:842–846
Fujisaki J, Masuda K, Ohmasa R, Akiba H, Miyamoto K, Hachiya K, Okuwaki S, Arai
  Y, Ichinose M, Suzuki H (1993) Endosonographic diagnosis of the depth of early
  gastric carcinoma with a sonoprobe system (20 MHz). Endosc Dig 5:157
Hiki Y (1991) Endoscopic treatment for gastric cancer from the surgical perspective.
  Gastroenterol Endosc 5:159
Hisamichi S, Sugawara N (1984) Mass screening for gastric cancer by x-ray examina-
  tion. Jpn J Clin Oncol 14:211-223
Jones DB, Guo LW, Reinhard MK, Soper NJ, Philpott GW, Connett J, Fleshman JW
  (1995) Impact of pneumoperitoneum on trocar site implantation of colon cancer in
  hamster model. Dis Colon Rectum 38:1182–1188
Kida M, Imaizumi H, Nishiyama K, Sada M, Shinomiya Y, Masuda H, Yoda S, Imamura

K, Sajima Y, Yamada Y, Sakaguchi T, Kobayashi K, Noto M, Saigenji K (1993) Usefulness of radial type ultrasonic probe for diagnosing upper gastrointestinal diseases. Endosc Dig 5:149

Kurihara N, Kubota T, Otani Y, Ohgami M, Kumai K, Sugiura H, Kitajima M (1998) Lymph node metastasis of early gastric cancer with submucosal invasion. Br J Surg 85:835–839

Ohashi S (1995) Laparoscopic intraluminal (intra-gastric) surgery for early gastric cancer: a new concept in laparoscopic surgery. Surg Endosc 9:169–171

Ohgami M, Kumai K, Otani Y, Wakabayashi G, Kubota T, Kitajima M (1994a) Laparoscopic wedge resection of the stomach for early gastric cancer using a lesion-lifting method. Dig Surg 11:64

Ohgami M, Watanabe M, Otani Y, Wakabayashi G, Kitajima M (1994b) Laparoscopic surgery for disease of digestive tract. Jpn J Endourol ESWL 7:144

Ohgami M, Kitajima M (1995) Combined laparoscopic and endoscopic excision of gastric mucosal lesions. In: Phillips EH, Rosenthal RJ (eds) Operative strategies in laparoscopic surgery. Springer, Berlin Heidelberg New York, pp. 141–145

Ohgami M, Otani Y, Kumai K, Kubota T, Kim YI, Kitajima M (1999) Curative laparoscopic surgery for early gastric cancer: five years experience. World J Surg 23:187–193

Otani Y, Murayama Y, Kurihara N, Kurihara N, Sakurai Y, Hoshiya Y, Yoshida M, Hayashi N, Ishizuka H, Ohgami M, Kubota T, Kumai K, Kitajima M, Sugino Y (1995) Analysis of 1,000 gastrectomies for early gastric cancer experienced in Keio University Hospital. The implication for therapeutic strategy. In: Nishi M, Sugano H, Takahashi T (eds) 1st International gastric cancer congress. Monduzzi Editore, Bologna, pp. 363–366

Tada M, Higaki S, Matsumoto Y, Ryo S, Karita M, Yanai H, Okita K (1993) Strip biopsy: its problems and measures implied by a long-term follow-up study (simultaneous and metachronous multiple cancers). Stomach and Intestine 28:1441

Thomas WM, Eaton MC, Hewett PJ (1996) A proposed model for the movement of cells within the abdominal cavity during CO_2 insufflation and laparoscopy. Aust N Z J Surg 66:105–106

Wexner SD, Cohen SM (1995) Port site metastases after laparoscopic colorectal surgery for cure of malignancy. Br J Surg 82:295–298

Whelan RL, Sellers GJ, Allendorf JD, Laird D, Bessler MD, Nowygrod R, Treat MR (1996) Trocar site recurrence is unlikely to result from aerosolization of tumor cells. Dis Colon Rectum 39:S7–13

CHAPTER 9

Laparoscopic Gastric Resection and Gastrectomy

E. Bärlehner

Introduction

Among laparoscopic operations of the stomach, the classic distal resections according to Billroth I and II, as well as total gastrectomy, currently occupy a modest place in the specialist literature. For this situation, three essential causes are evident: the high degree of laparoscopic difficulty, the decline in gastric resections in cases of benign illnesses, and the as yet unclarified influence of laparoscopic intervention in cases of carcinoma.

Development was initiated in 1992 by Goh et al. (1992) with a laparoscopic gastric resection according to Billroth II. The first laparoscopic gastric resection according to Billroth I was reported by Bärlehner et al. in 1994. In 1996, the first report of a laparoscopic gastrectomy for carcinoma followed (Ablassmeier et al. 1996a).

Small case series of laparoscopic gastric resections in cases of benign fundamental illness confirmed operative practicability (Ablassmeier et al. 1994; Fowler and White 1996; Geis et al. 1996; Mayers and Orebaugh 1998), just as it had been practicable in a standardized way in animal models (Moriya et al. 1997) and in cadavers (Ablassmeier et al. 1996b).

The first successful case reports on laparoscopic gastric resections and gastrectomies in cases of carcinoma (Bärlehner et al. 1994; Ballesta-Lopez et al. 1996; Choi et al. 1996; Kuo et al. 1998), according to oncosurgical rules with omentectomy and lymphadenectomy, permit the prediction of developments such as we are currently seeing in laparoscopic surgery for colorectal carcinoma.

The operations are practicable, carry no greater risk of complications, and have oncological radicality vis-à-vis open surgery (Bärlehner 1999; Ballesta-Lopez et al. 1996; Choi et al. 1996). In the majority of reports, the benefits obtained through rapid convalescence, less pain, and better cosmetic results are emphasized (Goh et al. 1997).

The general advantages of this minimally invasive technique appear to justify its application in resectional gastric surgery. The standardization of the laparoscopic operative procedure takes priority here. In cases of benign illness with partial gastric resection, the technical details, including safe skeletization and anastomosis, are of great importance. Here, total laparoscopic resection according to Billroth I or II is favored. Newer aspects of gastric resection in cases of early carcinoma in the form of "wedge resection" (Buyske et al. 1997; Dempsey et al. 1997), open up perspectives on laparoscopically extended gastrectomies. The general requirements in more advanced tumor stages with gastrectomy and D2 lymphadenectomy represent a great challenge for laparoscopy. The extreme difficulties on the technical operative side in cases of en-bloc resectioning are reflected in the lack of standardization in the case reports to date. Oncosurgical aspects require particular attention with regard to tumor cell dissemination, port metastases, and critical pathohistological expertise. Ultimately, only long-term study results will permit a final evaluation; but impressive problem-free courses of convalescence following laparoscopic surgery are already signaling a hopeful trend.

A 44-year-old female patient underwent a laparoscopic multivisceral gastrectomy for a highly malignant T-cell non-Hodgkin's lymphoma (gastric maltoma). The monoblock gastrectomy with D2 lymphadenectomy was combined with a partial left resection of the liver, left resection of the pancreas, and splenectomy. The patient was able to take a walk in the ward corridor on the second postoperative day, and could be released from hospital on the eighth postoperative day, completely free of complaints.

The Technique of Laparoscopic Partial and Total Gastric Resection

The patient is placed in a modified lithotomy (dorsosacral) position on the operating table. The leg supports are conjoined with a cross-board, on which the patient supports himself in a sitting posture; a 45° angling of the table is possible under these circumstances. Access to the proximal stomach is thus optimal. The operator stands between the patient's legs, an assistant is positioned to the right. Two monitors, placed right and left cranially, enable optimal collaboration on the part of all participants.

In our opinion, a high-flow insufflator and an UltraCision (Ethicon, Germany) tool, along with the additional monitor, are absolutely neces-

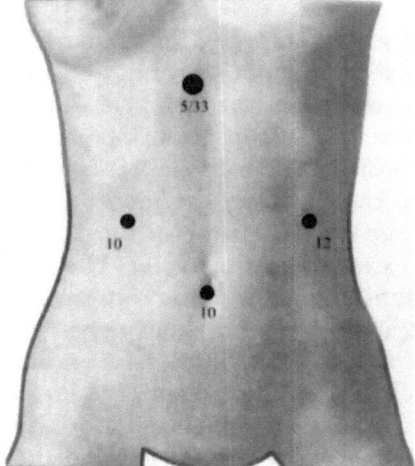 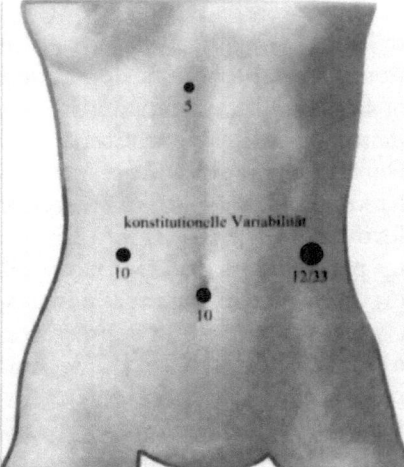

Fig. 9.1. Trocar position during Billroth I   **Fig. 9.2.** Trocar position during gastrectomy

sary special technical equipment. The operator should possess thorough knowledge of and skill in the entire spectrum of gastric surgery, and should have mastered conventional techniques perfectly. The degree of operative difficulty is clearly greater than that of laparoscopic colorectal surgery. Above-average skill in laparoscopic techniques is thus a requirement. The operation commences with the placement of a Veress needle in the upper navel area. A 10-mm optic trocar is then introduced through this incision. We use 30° angle optics as an optical system. At the same level or a little more cranially, two further trocars are placed, at one hand's width laterally right (10-mm trocar) and left (12-mm trocar). A 5-mm trocar in the epigastric angle guides the retraction rod. Depending on the extent of resection, the 5-mm trocar (Billroth I) or the 12-mm trocar (gastrectomy) is replaced by a 33-mm trocar (stapler) (Figs. 9.1 and 9.2).

Procedure When Carrying Out Distal Two-Thirds to Three-Quarters Resection According to Billroth I

Skeletization in cases of definitely benign fundamental illness is started at the Mikulicz point, at the side of the greater curvature. The gastrocolic ligament can be divided near the gastric wall without problem using UltraCision scissors (Fig. 9.3). When skeletizing proximally through the

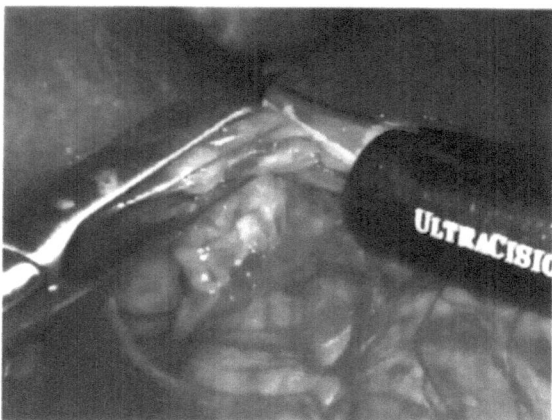

Fig. 9.3. Skeletization with the UltraCision

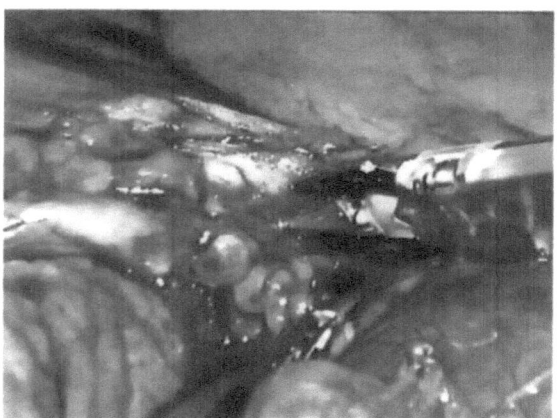

Fig. 9.4. Severance of vessels between clips

gastrolienal ligament, care must be taken that arterial perfusion through the short gastric and right gastroepiploic arteries is preserved. Preparation in the area of the stomach exit is preceded by Kocher's mobilization of the duodenum. This is a prerequisite of later tension-free anastomosis. Sectioning of the right gastroepiploic artery aids in avoiding hemorrhaging complications (Fig. 9.4). On the side of the lesser curvature, the common hepatic artery can easily be identified after sectioning of the Pars flaccida of the lesser omentum; in the further course, the gastroduodenal and right gastric arteries can also be identified. The latter is sectioned between clips. Depending upon the localization of the tumor, the lesser curvature can be skeletized near the wall, or, if the tumor is located on the lesser curvature side, the left gastric artery can be sectioned off between clips close to the stem. Cross-sectioning of the proximal stomach is carried out with a 60-mm linear cutter (Ethicon Endo-Surgery) instrument (18-mm trocar) or with smaller cutters applied repeatedly (Fig. 9.5). The portion of stomach folded out to the right renders the dorsal mobilization of the proximal duodenum easier. As a rule, this can be removed with a 30-mm cutter (Fig. 9.6). The removed gastric specimen is placed within a salvage sac. The tobacco-pouch suture at the duodenum can be carried out by means of a tobacco-pouch suturing instrument (Fig. 9.7), or by hand suture after resection of the clip suture closure (Fig. 9.8). We prefer the latter method. After introduction of the 33-mm trocar into the epigastric angle, the 25 or 28 airtight circular stapler, ILC 25 or 28 mm (Ethicon), is introduced and the compression plate is

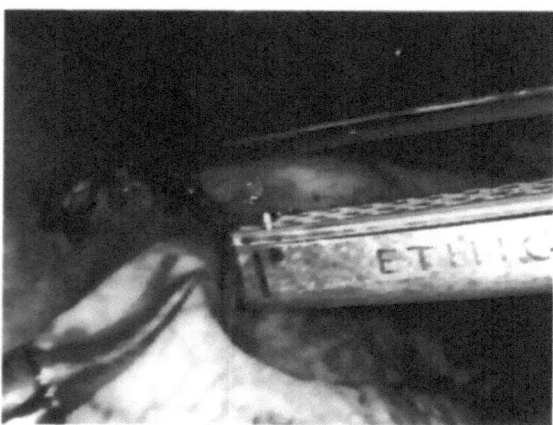

Fig. 9.5. Proximal gastric section

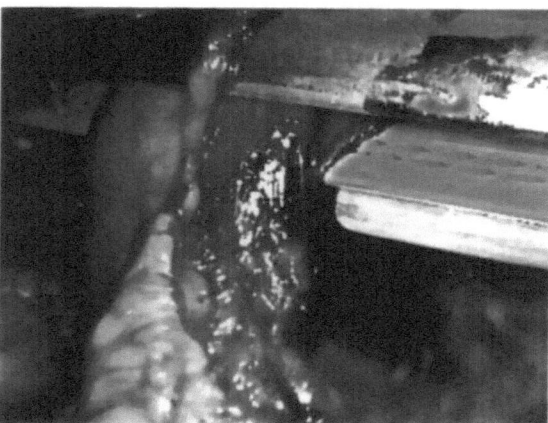

Fig. 9.6. Sectioning of duodenum

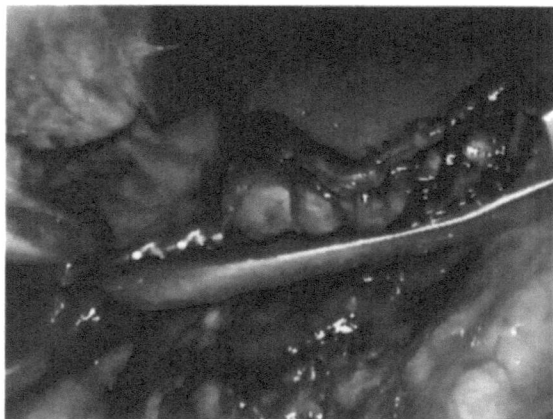

Fig. 9.7. Tobacco-pouch suture on the duodenal stump with tobacco-pouch suture clamp

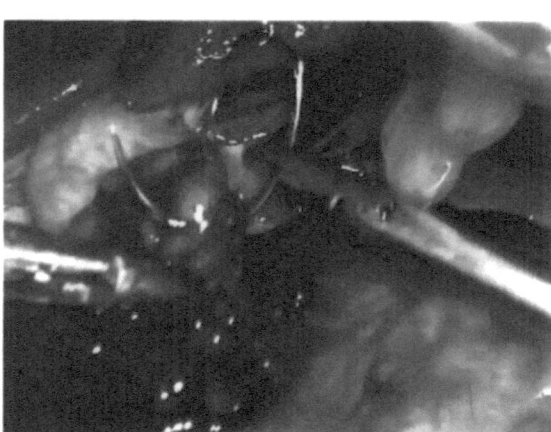

Fig. 9.8. Tobacco-pouch suture by hand on the duodenal stump

removed to a distance. The stapler head is placed within the duodenal stump, which occasionally results in handling difficulties (Fig. 9.9). After the tobacco-pouch suture has been fastened, the stapler shaft is disconnected. We then make an incision in the frontal wall of the gastric stump, using the UltraCision scissors (Fig. 9.10). We introduce the stapler shaft through this small gastrotomy into the stomach (Fig. 9.11). The row of clip sutures is perforated with the central spike at the point of transition to the greater curvature. After connection with the head portion (Fig. 9.12), anastomosis is carried out under close visual control and tension of the anastomosis must be avoided (Fig. 9.13). After the stapler is removed (Figs. 9.14, 9.15), the gastrotomy is closed using intracorpo-

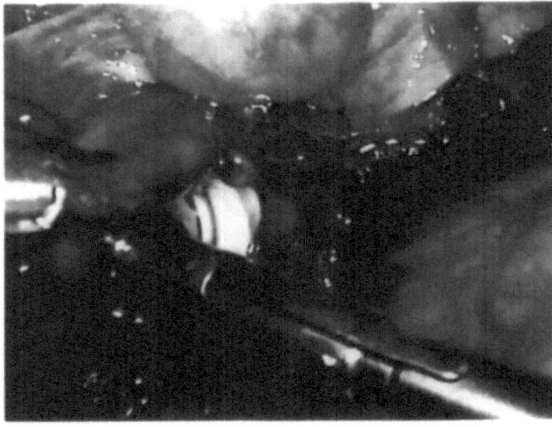

Fig. 9.9. Introduction of the stapler head into the duodenal stump

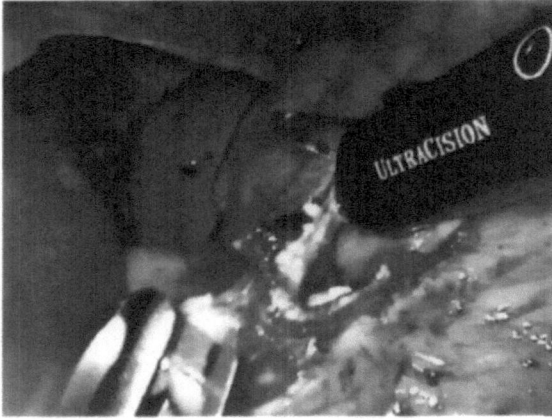

Fig. 9.10. Gastrotomy in the proximal gastric stump

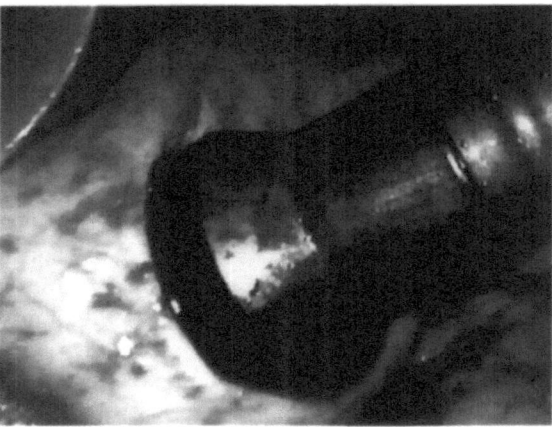

Fig. 9.11. Intraluminal stapler Endopath (Ethicon Endo-Surgery) in the gastric stump

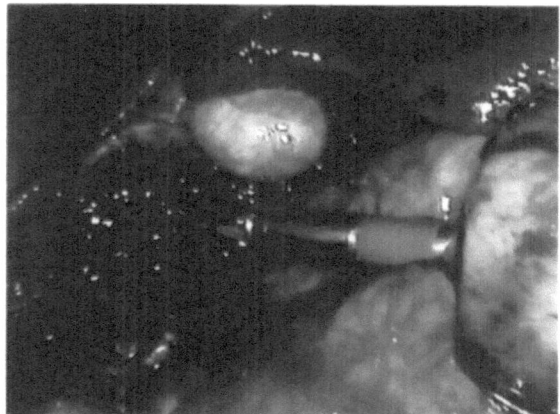

Fig. 9.12. Connection of the stapler and compression plate

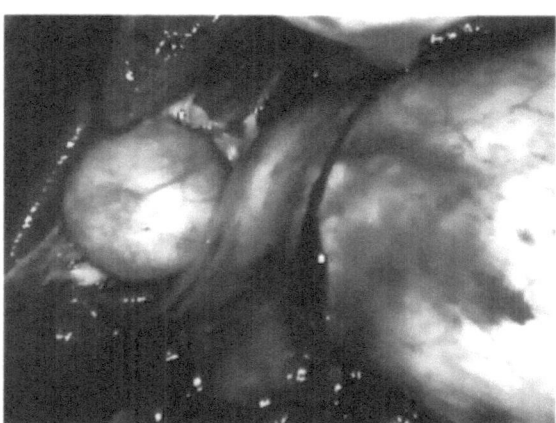

Fig. 9.13. Anastomosis

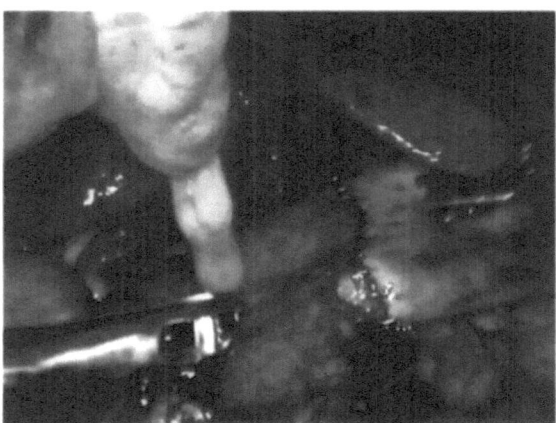

Fig. 9.14. Completed anastomosis

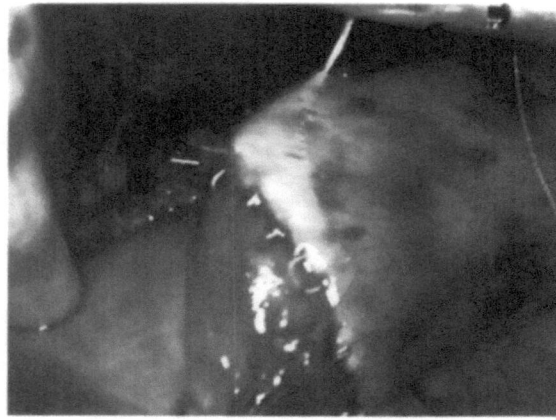

Fig. 9.15. Securing the anastomosis

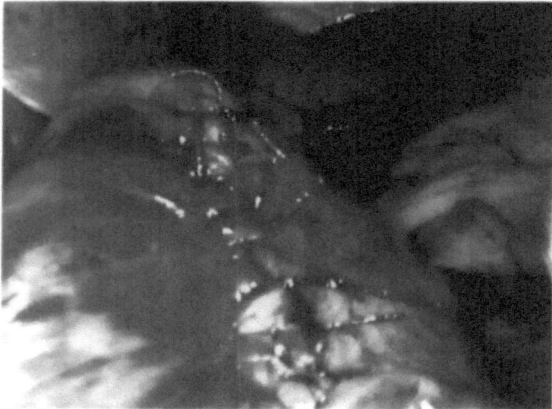

Fig. 9.16. Closing off the gastrotomy

rally fastened button sutures (Fig. 9.16). The tightness of the sutures and the anastomosis is checked by filling the stomach with methylene blue. Salvage of the resectate is carried out by means of the 33-mm trocar canal, widened if necessary. The operation is finished with drainage of the subhepatic space.

Operative Procedure in Cases of Gastric Carcinoma

The operative procedure in cases of gastric carcinoma is basically subject to oncosurgical laws. It starts with the detachment of the greater omentum from the transverse colon (Fig. 9.17). Conserving the spleen, the gastrolienal ligament is divided with truncal displacement of the right gastroepiploic artery. By pulling at the pylorus, the gastroduodenal artery and vein tense infrapylorically. Along with the lymph node, regularly recognizable here, both vessels are displaced between clips (Fig. 9. 18). Dissection of the hepatoduodenal ligament displays the choledochus, the hepatic artery, and the portal vein. The right gastric artery is

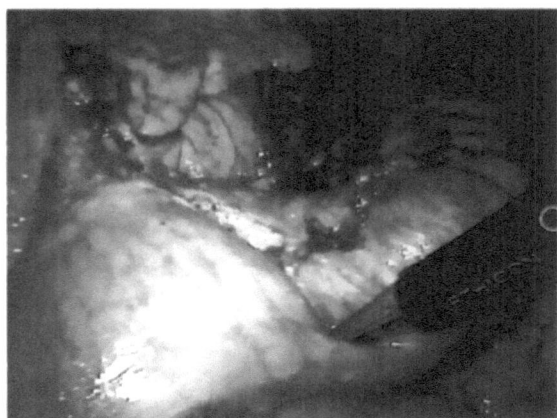

Fig. 9.17. Detachment of the greater omentum from the transverse colon

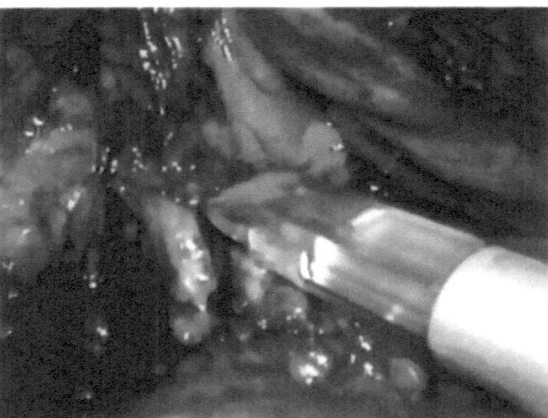

Fig. 9.18. Sectioning of the vessels between clips (gastroduodenal artery and vein)

sectioned between clips. By means of the lymphadenectomy along the common hepatic artery, which is to be laid free, the celiac trunk is reached (Fig. 9.19). Celiac lymphadenectomy is ancillary to the isolation of the left gastric artery and the splenic artery. The left gastric artery is closed off with an Absoloc clip (Ethicon) and displaced truncally (Fig. 9.20). The gastric coronary vein, which runs immediately adjacent to this region, is sectioned between metal clips. Complete detachment of the lesser omentum at the liver leads to the esophageal hiatus. By laying free both sides of the hiatus, the esophagus is isolated and both vagus stems are severed (Fig. 9.21). Finally, the monoblock preparation is fixed only at the duodenum and the esophagus. Postpylorically, the duodenum is displaced with a linear cutter (35 or 30 mm) (Fig. 9.22). Proxi-

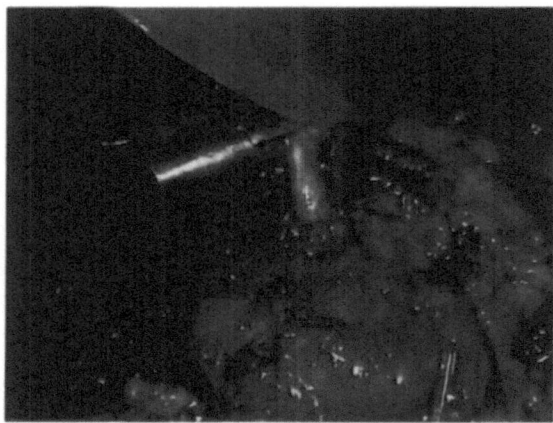

Fig. 9.19. Celiac trunk

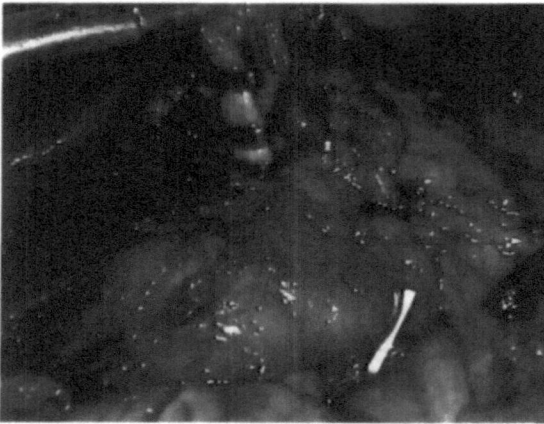

Fig. 9.20. Clipped left gastric artery and gastric coronary vein

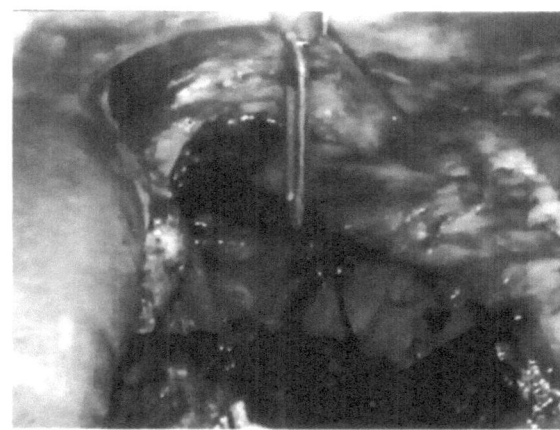

Fig. 9.21. Diaphragmatic shank and isolated esophagus

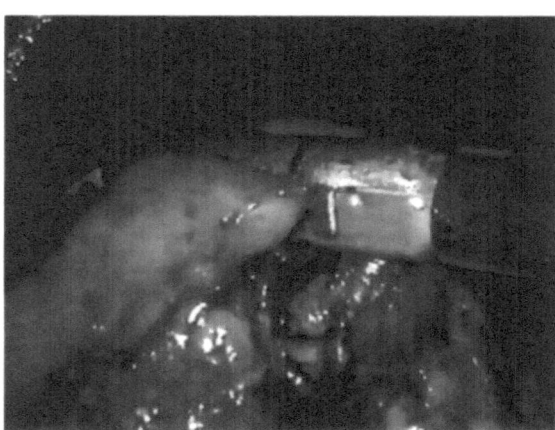

Fig. 9.22. Sectioning of the duodenum

mally, displacement to the esophagus or as a near-total gastrectomy with a gastric portion of maximum 3 cm in length is carried out, depending upon the location and entity of the tumor. The preparation is transferred to a salvage sac. After resectioning of the clip suture row on the esophagus or in the portion of gastric wall involved, a tobacco-pouch suture is laid using monophile suturing and a needle-carrier (Fig. 9.23). After exchanging the 12-mm trocar at the left costal arch with a 33-mm trocar, the gastight circular stapler (25 mm) is introduced (ILC-Ethicon Endo-Surgery). The compression plates are removed to a distance and the head is introduced into the esophagus or the gastric cuff (Fig. 9.24). The tobacco-pouch suture is tied intracorporally. The stapler is then disconnected and the shaft removed. Now, the proximal loop of the jejunum is

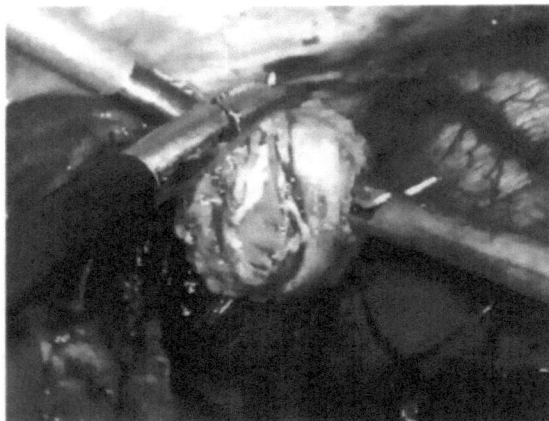

Fig. 9.23. Tobacco-pouch suture on the esophagus

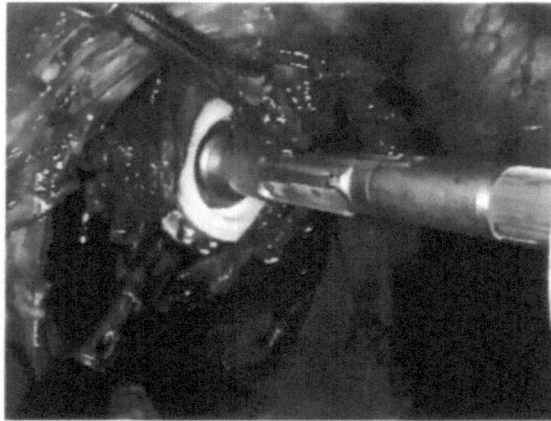

Fig. 9.24. Compression plate in the esophagus

located and the duodenal flexure is identified with certainty. The envisaged loop is tested for its length to the anastomosis and the planned location of the enteroanastomosis is marked and fixed in a clamp. The 33-mm trocar is removed and the trocar canal is secured with a ring foil. Luxation of the salvage sac and removal of the resectate follow. The intestinal clamp, together with the jejunum, is now led to the mini-laparotomy and the intestine is guided to the outside. A typical open sectioning and placement of the Roux-en-Y anastomosis using a one-row extramucosal suture technique, while excluding a 40–45-cm long Roux shank, is carried out. The stapler shaft is now passed through the 33-mm trocar and then transferred into the open Roux shank. In order to prevent the intestine from slipping away, it is fixed to the shaft by means of a thick ligature. Thereupon, repositioning of the intestine and the stapler is accomplished by the mini-lap., and the 33-mm trocar being thrust after ensures restoration of a sealed, gastight situation. Perforation of the intestine with the central spike (crutch anastomosis) and connection to the compression plate (Fig. 9.25) are then performed under laparoscopic conditions. Anastomosis is carried out with optimal visual control. After severing the support thread at the stapler shaft, the stapler is removed and the anastomosis rings are checked. Using the linear cutter, the "crutch end" is displaced and closed off (Fig. 9.26). We always fix the anastomosis in hiatus with the intracorporally fastened button sutures, thus granting the anastomosis additional relief from tension. The placement of a feeding tube in the lower Roux section can be controlled well.

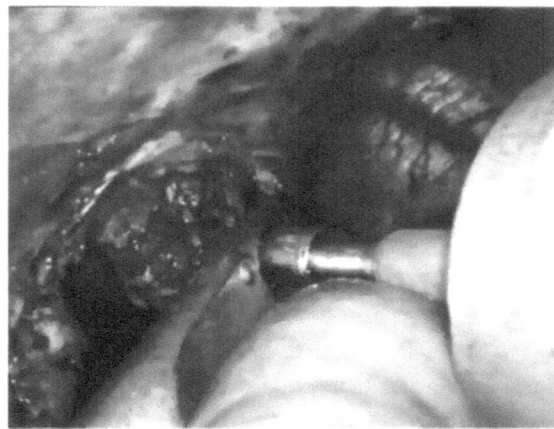

Fig. 9.25. Connecting the stapler

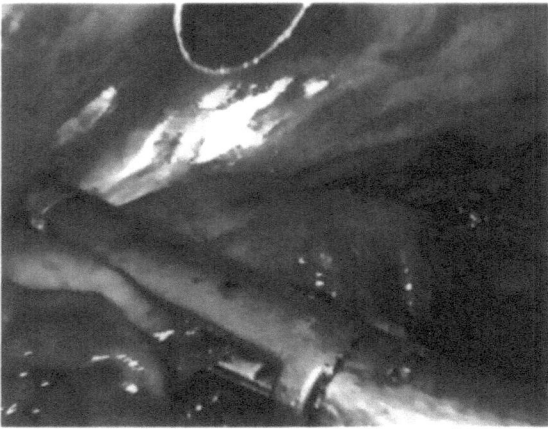

Fig. 9.26. Closing off of the "crutch end"

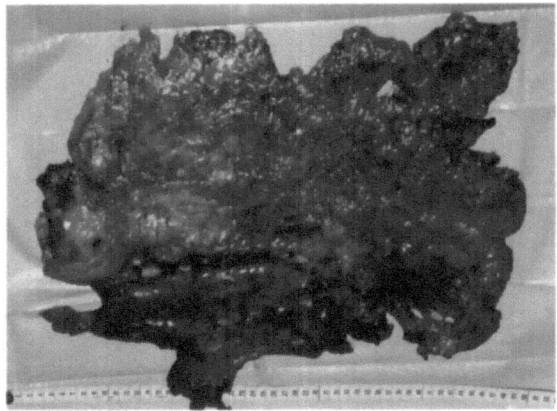

Fig. 9.27. Monoblock resectate

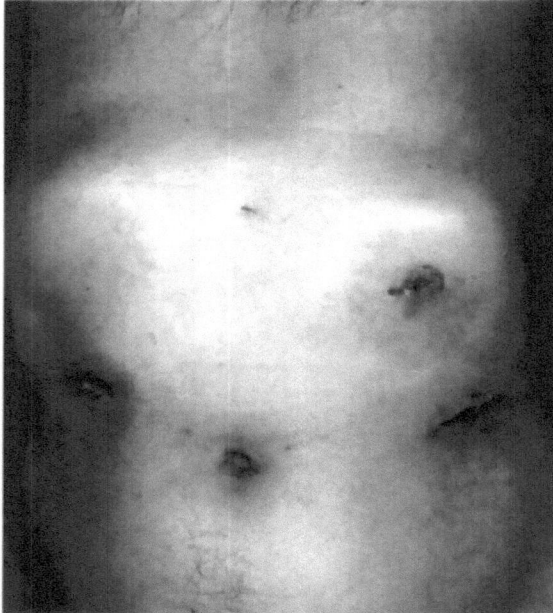

Fig. 9.28. Postoperative abdominal view

The operation is completed with drainage of the subhepatic space and the lesser pelvis. The monoblock resectate and the postoperative abdominal view are shown in Figs. 9.27 and 9.28, respectively.

Patients

In the period between May 1993 to December 1998, 260 laparoscopic gastric operations altogether were carried out at the Klinikum Buch. For 17 patients, it was a matter of classic resectioning procedures. Seven patients presented with a benign illness: two cases with gastric ulcer, one with duodenal ulcer, and four with gastrointestinal stromal tumor. The

Table 9.1. Laparoscopic gastric resection in cases of benign fundamental illness (n=7)

Patient	Age	Sex	Diagnosis	Operative technique	Duration (min)	Complications	Advantageous outcome
1	52	F	Gastric ulcer	Billroth I	290	0	+
2	74	F	GIST	Billroth I	270[a]	0	+
3	73	F	GIST	Billroth I	195	0	+
4	68	F	GIST	Billroth I	280	0	+
5	64	F	Gastric ulcer	Billroth I	190	0	+
6	35	M	Duodenal ulcer	Billroth I	240	0	+
7	75	M	GIST	Billroth II	250	0	+

[a] With cholecystectomy and ovarectomy.

Table 9.2. Laparoscopic gastric resection (GR) in cases of malignant fundamental illness (*n*=10)

Patient	Age	Sex	Diagnosis	Operative technique	Duration (min)	Complications	Advantageous outcome
1	81	F	Adenocarcinoma	Subtotal GR Billroth I	240	0	+
2	66	F	Maltoma	Gastrectomy	230	0	+
3	58	M	Adenocarcinoma	Gastrectomy	280	0	+
4	76	F	Adenocarcinoma	Gastrectomy	330	0	+
5	68	F	Adenocarcinoma	Gastrectomy	325	0	+
6	82	M	Adenocarcinoma	Gastrectomy	340	+[a]	+
7	65	M	Adenocarcinoma	Gastrectomy	345	0	+
8	70	M	Adenocarcinoma	Gastrectomy	210	0	+
9	44	F	T-cell NHL	Gastrectomy, multi-visceral	300	0	+
10	80	M	Adenocarcinoma	gastrectomy	290	0	+

NHL, non-Hodgkin's lymphoma.
[a] Relaparotomy first day following operation due to duodenal clamp suture leakage.

five women and two men were between the ages of 35 and 74. In six cases, a laparoscopic resection according to Billroth I was carried out, in one case according to Billroth II (Table 9.1). Ten patients were operated for malignant illnesses (Table 9.2). In eight of these, the malignancy was an adenocarcinoma, in two, a little-differentiated maltoma presented. The five women and five men were between the ages of 44 and 82. In nine cases, laparoscopically-assisted gastrectomy was carried out, and in one a totally laparoscopic subtotal gastric resection according to Billroth I was carried out. All patients underwent a preoperative gastroscopy with biopsy and a sonography. In the case of histological confirmation of carcinoma, the diagnostic procedures were extended through the addition of endosonography and computed tomography (CT). In the case of one female patient, the diagnosis of gastric carcinoma was made in the course of a laparoscopic colon operation. Postoperative gastroscopy and biopsy could not confirm the diagnosis. CT and endosonography merely displayed the thickening of the wall in the antrum. Relaparoscopy histologically confirmed the gastric carcinoma.

The duration of operations ranged between 190 and 290 min (on average 245 min) for partial gastric resection and benign fundamental illness, whereby in one case cholecystectomy and ovarectomy were carried out synchronically. All seven patients showed complication-free postoperative courses. In the case of laparoscopically-assisted gastrectomies with D2 lymphadenectomy, the duration of operations ranged between 240 and 340 min (on average 290 min). Extended operations were carried out in the cases of three patients – cholecystectomy, transversum resection, and, in one case, a partial resection of the liver with left pancreatectomy and splenectomy. As regards postoperative complications, duodenal stump insufficiency was observed in only one patient, which

Table 9.3. Laparoscopic gastric resection in cases of malignant illness (n=10)

Pathohistological evaluation
pT2 pN0 (0/24) M0 L0 V0 G3 R0
Non-Hodgkin lymphoma (maltoma) 0/42
pT1 pN0 (0/34) M0 L0 V0 G3 R0
pT3 pN0 (0/17) M0 L1 V2 G3 – 4 R0
pT3 pN0 (0/25) M0 L0 V0 G3 R0[a]
pT1 pN0 (0/25) M0 L0 V0 G3 R0
pT1 pN0 (0/73) M0 L0 V0 G2 R0
pT1pN0 (0/33) M0 L0 V0 G2 R0
pT2pN0 (0/34) M0 L0 V0 G2 R0
Non-Hodgkin lymphoma 0/28

[a] Omental tumor with the same histology.

was laparoscopically revised on the first postoperative day by means of restapling. The further course of recovery remained free of complications.

The histological evaluation is reproduced in Table 9.3. By means of subtle processing, a Ro resection was documented in all patients. In the case of female patient No.° 5, this must be modified slightly, insofar as an omental metastasis in the gastrocolic ligament was diagnosed intraoperatively and was treated by means of en-bloc omentectomy. Histologically, this finding was evaluated as an isolated omental metastasis.

Evaluation

Partial gastric resection and total gastrectomy can be carried out laparoscopically. It is foreseeable that the controversy surrounding laparoscopic oncosurgery will escalate anew with the inclusion of gastric tumors. On the other hand, it must be assumed that oncosurgical precision can be guaranteed in analogy to colorectal tumor surgery (Bärlehner 1999; Bärlehner et al. 1998; Böhm et al. 1997; Franklin et al. 1995; Kökkerling et al. 1997; Kuthe et al. 1996). Adhering to oncosurgical principles in cases of gastric carcinoma (Böttcher et al. 1994; Siewert et al. 1996) must take priority as the most important principle of laparoscopic gastric surgery. Recent publications on local excision in the case of T_1 tumor and low malignancy (Namieno et al 1996; Yoshida et al. 1997) are only exceptionally possible in cases with mucosessile tumors, according to Hermanek (1996). The currently valid standard is radical resection including radical lymphadenectomy (D2 dissection). These principles were adhered to in the cases of all of our patients, and the stomach, together with the omentum and the lymph nodes of the second compartment, were resected en bloc and saved.

The independent histological processing of the resection preparations was executed in accordance with the criteria of the UICC (1993). The required lymph node number for a pNo finding of 15 was fulfilled in all resectates. On average, 34 lymph nodes were found in our preparations. The monoblock principle was adhered to in all cases; tumor injuries or other iatrogenic tumor cell dissemination could not be detected. In all patients, an Ro resection was achieved. The histologic evaluation is reproduced in Table 9.3. In eight cases, an adenocarcinoma was present (four intestinal type, four diffuse type), and in two cases a highly malignant maltoma was present.

The follow-up checks on our patients have hitherto revealed no dissemination, local relapses, nor metastases of the trocar channels. The average duration of observation was 10 months (3 – 37 months).

As regards operative technique, good general view and microdissection with magnification are two features of particular value. The advantages of minimalization of blood loss and abdominal wall trauma, together with low peritoneal trauma, which have been repeatedly described, are regularly reproducible. To what extent immunologically positive effects are attainable, and relevant for the patient, must remain an open question for the time being. The early effect of laparoscopic advantages is subjectively persuasive. Early mobility, minimal postaggression syndrome, rapid functionality of the intestine (peristalsis on the first postoperative day), no pulmonary complications, less pain, better cosmetic results, and no wound-healing problems are all convincing. The technical effort required, together with the requisite laparoscopic skills in the highest degree represent a problem. The amount of training needed for a completely standardized course of the operation is far greater than in the case of colorectal operations. But our most recent experience has confirmed a clear learning effect here, too, with a drastic reduction of the time required. The execution of this demanding operation with only *one* assistant is an advantage.

Gastric resection in cases of benign fundamental illness is an excellent method. Applying our standardized distal resection according to Billroth I, the operation can be carried out completely laparoscopically. The indication for gastric resection need very rarely be posited nowadays, which greatly prolongs any training effect. Nonetheless, the advantages of the minimally invasive procedure since our first Billroth I resection (Goh et al. 1997) have been regularly reproducible.

A general spread of laparoscopic gastric resection or gastrectomy cannot be predicted on the basis of the literature to date. Only a few case reports and small series have been published (Ballesta-Lopez et al 1996; Choi et al. 1996; Fowler and White 1996; Geis et al. 1996; Kuo et al. 1998) since the first reports (Ablassmeier et al. 1996a; Bärlehner et al. 1994; Goh et al. 1992). The agreement of our results with those of Choi and coworkers (1996) is given (Table 9.4). Goh et al. (1997) presented an international survey of 16 surgeons with 118 laparoscopic gastric resections. The distribution of the resection procedure demonstrates the degree of difficulty: 11 Billroth I, 87 Billroth II, 10 antrectomies with vagotomy, 10 total gastrectomies. Of the 16 surgeons, ten evaluated the operation as more advantageous than the open procedure. For four surgeons, the operation was too difficult and took too much time, while two surgeons were uncertain in evaluating the advantages over an open operation.

Table 9.4. Comparison of the literature on laparoscopic gastrectomy

Reference	Number of patients	OP Duration (min)	Number of lymph nodes
Choi et al. 1996	6	340	22.5
Bärlehner et al. 1998	7	295	34

For the present, laparoscopic gastric resection will remain a privilege of a few laparoscopic all-round surgeons.

In summary, it is foreseeable that laparoscopic gastric resection will gain in significance in the future. Both partial and total gastric resection are technically possible and can be carried out excellently under standardized conditions. In cases of malignant fundamental illnesses, laparoscopic subtotal or total gastrectomies with radical D2 lymphadenectomy are also possible under adherence to all oncosurgical principles. Surgically and histologically, the same radicality can be attained as in open procedures. The profit lies in lower complication rates and functional advantages. For definitive evaluation, we must await future results.

References

Ablassmeier B, Steinhilper U, Bandl WD, Ziehen T, Munster W, Fockersperger H (1994) 100 Jahre nach Billroth. Laparoskopische distale Magenresektion Billroth I und Billroth II. Chirurg 65(4):367–372

Ablassmeier B, Gellert K, Said S, Tanzella U, Müller JM (1996a) Laparoskopische Gastrektomie. Eine Fallbeschreibung. Chirurg 67:643–647

Ablassmeier B, Gellert K, Tanzella U, Müller JM (1996b) Laparoscopie Billroth II gastrectomy. J Laparoendosc Surg 6(5):319–324

Ballesta-Lopez C, Bastida-Vila X, Catarci M, Mato R, Ruggiero R (1996) Laparoscopic Billroth II distal subtotal gastrectomy with gastric stump suspension for gastric malignancies. Am J Surg 171(2):289–292

Bärlehner E (1999) Erste Erfahrungen mit der laparoskopischen Magenresektion bei benignen und malignen Tumoren. Zentralbl Chir 124:346–350

Bärlehner E, Schwetling R, Anders S, Mau H (1994) Laparoskopische Magenresektion nach Billroth I. MIC 1:7–9

Bärlehner E, Heukrodt B, Anders S (1998) Laparoskopische Rektumchirurgie beim Karzinom. Zentralbl Chir 123:1164–1168

Böhm B, Schwenk W, Gründel K, Junghans T, Müller JM (1997) Die Bedeutung der laparoskopischen Technik beim primaren colorectalen Carcinom. Chirurg 68:231–236

Böttcher K, Siewert JR, Roder JD, Busch R et al. (1994) Risiko der chirurgischen Therapie des Magencarcinoms in Deutschland. Ergebnisse der Deutschen Magencarcinom-Studie 1992. Chirurg 65:298

Buyske J, McDonald M, Fernandez C, Munson JL, Sanders LE, Tsao J, Birkett DH (1997) Minimally invasive management of low-grade and benign gastric tumors. Surg Endosc 11(11):1084–1087

Choi SH, Yoon DS, Chi HS, Min JS (1996) Laparoscopy-assisted radical subtotal gastrectomy for early gastric carcinoma. Yonsei Med J 37(3):174–180

Dempsey DT, Kelberman IA, Dabezies MA (1997) Laparoscopic resection of gastric leiomyosarcoma. J Laparoendosc Adv Surg Tech A7(6):357–362

Fowler DL, White SA (1996) Laparoscopic gastrectomy: five cases. Surg Laparosc Endosc 6(2):98–101

Franklin MW, Rosenthal D, Norem RF (1995) Prospective evaluation of laparoscopic colon resection versus open colon resection for adenocarcinoma – a multicenter study. Surg Endosc 9:811

Geis WP, Baxt R, Kim HC (1996) Benign gastric tumors. Minimally invasive approach. Surg Endosc 10(4):407–410

Goh PM, Tekant Y, Kum CK, Isaac J, Shang NS (1992) Totally intra-abdominal laparoscopy Billroth II gastrectomy. Surg Endosc 6:160–165

Goh PM, Alponat A, Mak K, Kurn CK (1997) Early international results of laparoscopic gastrectomies. Surg Endosc 11(6):650–652

Hermanek P (1996) Differenziertes chirurgisches Vorgehen bei der kurativen Therapie des Magenkarzinoms. Leber-Magen-Darm 26(2):67–72

Köckerling F, Reymond MA, Schneider C, Hohenberger W (1997) Fehler und Gefahren in der onkologischen laparoskopischen Chirurgie. Chirurg 68:215–224

Kuo WH, Lee WJ, Chen CN, Yuan RH, Yu SC (1998) Laparoscopic subtotal gastrectomy with lymphadenectomy in a patient with early gastric cancer. J Formos Med Assoc 97(2):127–130

Kuthe A, Faust H, Quast G, Reichel K (1996) Laparoskopische resektive Eingriffe bei kolorektalem Karzinom. MIC 5:2–5

Mayers TM, Orebaugh MG (1998) Totally laparoscopic Billroth I gastrectomy. J Am Coll Surg 186(1):100–103

Moriya H, Shimizu S, Okano T, Yamaguchi S (1997) Experimental study of laparoscopic gastrectomy: intracorporeal Billroth I gastroduodenostomy. Surg Laparosc Endosc 7(1):32–37

Namieno T, Koito K, Higashi T, Sato N, Uchino J (1996) General pattern of lymph node metastasis in early gastric carcinoma. World J Surg 20(8):996–1000

Siewert JR, Stein HJ, Böttcher K (1996) Lymphadenektomie bei Tumoren des oberen Gastrointestinaltrakts. Chirurg 67:877–888

UICC (1993) TNM supplement. In: Hermanek P, Henson DE, Hutter RVP, Sobin LH (eds) A commentary for uniform use. Springer, Berlin Heildelberg New York

Yoshida M, Otani Y, Ohgami M, Kubota T, Kumai K, Mukai M, Kitajima M (1997) Surgical management of gastric leiomyosarcoma: evaluation of the propriety of laparoscopic wedge resection. World J Surg 21(4):440–443

Subject Index

achalasia 35
β3-Adrenoceptor gene 64
amyloidosis 44
antacids 19
antireflux surgery
– indications 23
– contraindications 23
– techniques 23
– – 360° fundoplication 23
– complications 31
– results 33

barium esophagogram 11
barium swallow under fluoroscopy 41
Barrett's esophagus 1, 2, 8, 11
benzimidazoles 17
Billroth I 114
birds beak 42
body mass index (BMI) 62, 73
botulinum toxin injection 49
BTX see endoscopic botulinum toxin

calcium channel blockers 45
cardiomyotomy
– indications 56
– contraindications 56
– surgical technique 56
– complications 59
– results 59
Chagas' disease 35, 44
chest discomfort 38
chronic esophagitis 1
cisapride 18
Cushing's syndrome 64, 73

diaphanoscopy 31
dietary regimen 68
duodeno-gastric reflux 8
dysphagia 31, 35, 38

early gastric cancer surgery 97
– indications 98
– procedures 98
– advantages 109
– problems 109
Eder-Puestow guidewire 47
endoscopic botulinum toxin (BTX)
  injection 45
energy expenditure 67
epiphrenic diverticulum 42
esophageal acid clearance 5
esophageal bougienage 44
esophageal manometry 15, 42
esophageal mucosal resistance 7
esophageal perforation 48
esophageal pH-metry 13
esophagitis 2
esophagoscopy 9

flexible electrolaparoscope 89

„gas bloat" syndrome 31
gastrectomy 87, 112
– indication 88
– surgical technique 89
– results 95
gastric acid hypersecretion 8
gastric banding
– indications 73

– contraindications 73
– surgical technique 74
– complications 83
– results 85
gastric carcinoma 121
gastric emptying 7
gastric resection 112
gastroesophageal reflux disease
    (GERD) 1
– -associated symptoms 8
GERD see gastroesophageal reflux dis-
    ease

heartburn 1, 8
hemifundoplication (Toupet) 29
hiatus hernia 1, 4
high-grade dysplasia 11

intragastric mucosal resection 97, 104,
    105

leptin 61, 65
LES see lower esophageal sphincter
lesion-lifting method 97, 98
liver and spleen laceration 31
lower esophageal sphincter (LES) 2, 7,
    35
– dysfunction 3
– relaxation 36, 43
– resting tone 3
low-grade dysplasia 11
lymph node dissection 87, 90, 91, 92, 93

minimal paraesophageal dissection 29
mucosal gastric cancer 97
mucosal protective agents 19
MUSE classification 9, 10

NIDDM see non-insulin-dependent
    diabetes mellitus
Nissen fundoplication 33
nitrates 45
nocturnal regurgitation 35

noncardiac chest pain 35
non-insulin-dependent diabetes
    mellitus (NIDDM) 61, 65

obese (ob) gene 61, 65
obesity 61

paraesophageal herniation 31
partial and total gastric resection 113
perforation of the esophagus and
    stomach 31
pneumatic dilatation 46
pneumothorax 31
prokinetic agents 18
proton-pump inhibitors 17
pulmonary aspiration 38

recurrent reflux 33
reflux disease 10
reflux esophagitis 1, 10
regurgitation 38
Rigiflex dilator 46, 47

salivery function 6
Savary-Miller classification 9, 10
scleroderma 5
secondary achalasia 38
„slipped" Nissen syndrome 33
stomach perforation 83

tortuous megaesophagus 42
Toupet hemifundoplication 29

vasoactive intestinal polypeptide
    (VIP) 36

wedge resection of the stomach 98
weight loss 38

xerostomia 6

yield pressure 40